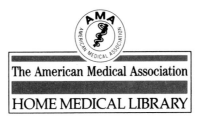

The American Medical Association

HOME MEDICAL LIBRARY

THE BRAIN AND NERVOUS SYSTEM

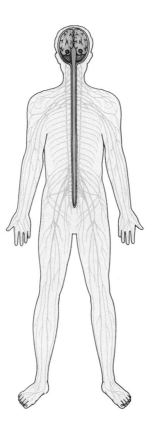

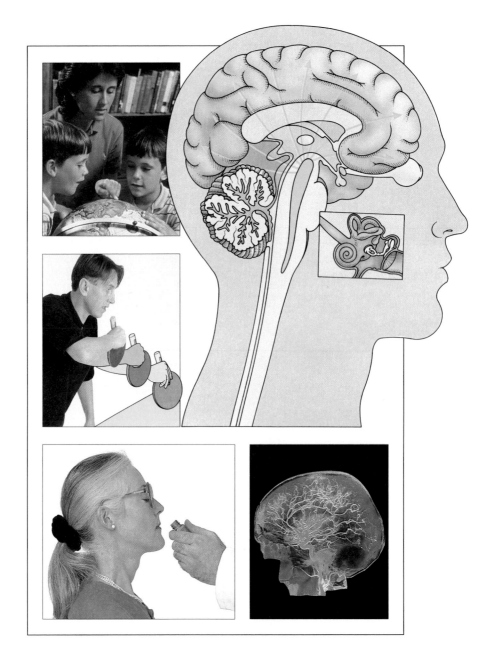

THE AMERICAN MEDICAL ASSOCIATION

THE BRAIN AND NERVOUS SYSTEM

Medical Editor
CHARLES B. CLAYMAN, MD

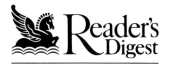

THE READER'S DIGEST ASSOCIATION, INC.
Pleasantville, New York/Montreal

Library of Congress Cataloging in Publication Data

The Brain and nervous system / the American Medical Association;
    medical editor, Charles B. Clayman.
        p. cm — (The American Medical Association home medical
    library)
    Includes index.
    ISBN 0-89577-396-1
    1. Brain — Physiology — Popular works. 2. Nervous system —
Physiology — Popular works. 3. Brain — Diseases — Popular works.
4. Nervous system — Diseases — Popular works. I. Clayman, Charles B.
II. American Medical Association. III. Series.
QP376.B6962 1991
612.8 — dc20   91-12825

FOREWORD

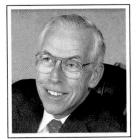

Every thought, every feeling, every act, and every bodily function in our lives is ruled by the large mass of nerve cells that we call the brain. Your brain works constantly to keep you warm, upright, and breathing. It also helps you perceive the outside world. Right now, for example, you are using millions of nerve cells to read and understand this page. Yet many of us know no more about the functioning of our brain than we do about the wiring system in a car or the computer we use at the office.

In this volume of the AMA Home Medical Library we present the brain, and the body's vast network of nerves, in terms that can be easily and immediately understood. We also provide a guide to brain and nervous system disorders. The opening chapter describes the overall purpose of a nervous system and its structure in our bodies. In later chapters, we explore the function of the brain, as it directs both those activities of which we are aware and those beneath our level of consciousness.

Nervous system and brain disorders affect a significant proportion of the population. These disorders range from conditions that can begin in childhood, such as epilepsy, to those neurological disorders most prevalent in the over-65 age group, such as stroke and Parkinson's disease. The final chapter in this volume examines some of the major brain and nervous system disorders and their symptoms, diagnosis, and treatment. A comprehensive glossary of medical terms will also help you understand the often complex terminology of the neurologist and neurosurgeon.

We at the American Medical Association hope this volume increases your understanding of the brain – the most sophisticated and incredible "living computer" in the world.

JAMES S. TODD, MD
Executive Vice President
American Medical Association

CONTENTS

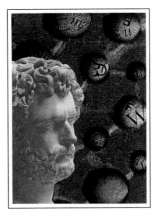

CHAPTER ONE

STRUCTURES AND SYSTEMS

INTRODUCTION

WHAT IS A NERVOUS SYSTEM?

EVOLUTION AND DEVELOPMENT

HOW IS THE NERVOUS SYSTEM ORGANIZED?

NERVE CELLS

THE BRAIN

THE SPINAL CORD AND PERIPHERAL NERVES

YOUR BRAIN and nervous system are the most important and complex parts of your body. They regulate your internal bodily functions and coordinate your responses to the outside environment. Your brain is the seat of your intelligence, memory, will, and emotion. Although your heart and liver can be replaced, your brain cannot. Even if it could, you would no longer be the same person.

We have only recently begun to understand the brain's central coordinating role and the workings of the nervous system. This understanding was impossible until medical science reached a fairly sophisticated stage of development. The ancient Greeks viewed the heart as the source of all higher functions. But an influential minority believed that the brain was the source of such experiences as thought, pleasure, pain, laughter, and fear.

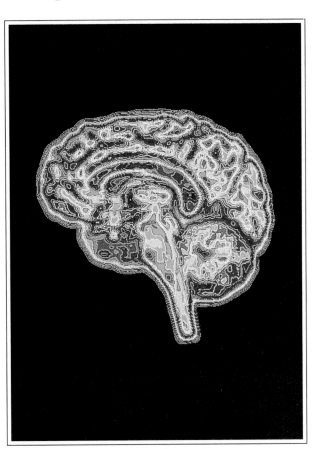

Some of the early Greek scientists supported their views with evidence gained from dissections of the brain and nervous system. Later, during the Renaissance, knowledge of the brain's structure flourished after Flemish physician and professor Vesalius (1514-1564) founded the science of anatomy. For the next 300 years, doctors learned much about the nature of nervous system diseases by observing the patterns of illness in disorders such as stroke. Using simple but meticulous observation, doctors described such conditions as Parkinson's disease, Huntington's chorea, and Down's syndrome. But detailed understanding of the underlying disease processes had to wait for advances in pathology. These advances included improvements in microscopes and in methods of staining and studying tissues taken from the nervous system.

By the beginning of this century, neurologists and neuroanatomists used these technical advances to reveal the complexity of the connections inside the brain and the detailed structure of individual nerve cells. These scientists not only studied disease but also learned much about normal brain function from studying people with brain disorders and from examining their brains after death. During the past 20 years, advanced imaging techniques and chemical studies of brain cells have improved our understanding of brain function dramatically. We have also learned much more about the way nerve cells transmit messages within the brain. Our knowledge of brain function is still far exceeded by what we do not know. But researchers today are making exciting new discoveries about the workings of the brain and nervous system.

WHAT IS A NERVOUS SYSTEM?

Your nervous system is an interconnected network of nerve cells, or neurons, that coordinates your actions. It senses the environment and helps you react to external stimuli by thinking, moving, and speaking. Your nervous system also regulates your internal, involuntary functions, such as breathing and heart rate. All nerve cells pass information from one part of your body to another. To perform this function, some of the nerve cells are elongated so that they can connect all parts of your body.

The simple reflex

A basic form of nervous system activity is the simple reflex. Reflex actions require a receptor to sense an incoming stimulus, a sensory nerve cell to carry the signal into the organism, and a junction (synapse) between the sensory nerve cell and a motor nerve cell, which then carries the signal to an organ, usually a muscle. Reflexes ensure that a stimulus triggers a particular response.

Simpler organisms have more elementary nervous systems. A simple animal such as a jellyfish, with a limited range of actions, possesses a nervous system that operates almost entirely by means of simple reflexes (see below). Through such a system, the jellyfish is able to avoid danger, such as a poisonous substance, or move toward desirable objects, such as food.

More advanced animals developed the ability to learn from previous experience. Because the simple reflex is too

A simple nervous system

The nervous system of a jellyfish consists of a circular network of nerve cells. Sensory input comes from tiny gravity-sensing organs called statocysts. The only responding organ is a circular swimming muscle, which moves the jellyfish through the water as it contracts.

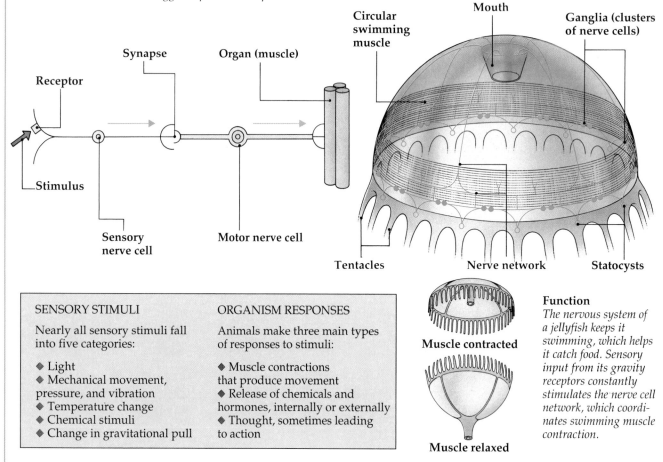

Receptor
Synapse
Organ (muscle)
Stimulus
Sensory nerve cell
Motor nerve cell

Circular swimming muscle
Mouth
Ganglia (clusters of nerve cells)
Tentacles
Nerve network
Statocysts

Muscle contracted
Muscle relaxed

Function
The nervous system of a jellyfish keeps it swimming, which helps it catch food. Sensory input from its gravity receptors constantly stimulates the nerve cell network, which coordinates swimming muscle contraction.

SENSORY STIMULI	ORGANISM RESPONSES
Nearly all sensory stimuli fall into five categories: ◆ Light ◆ Mechanical movement, pressure, and vibration ◆ Temperature change ◆ Chemical stimuli ◆ Change in gravitational pull	Animals make three main types of responses to stimuli: ◆ Muscle contractions that produce movement ◆ Release of chemicals and hormones, internally or externally ◆ Thought, sometimes leading to action

basic for this purpose, it must be augmented by an entire network of nerve cells that can analyze information from many sources, store the data, and coordinate the organism's responses. This network of nerve cells must allow or inhibit simple reflex action. In more advanced animals, these nerve cells group together into a central control center called a brain.

Surprisingly complex behavior can be organized by a relatively simple nervous system. Artificial animals that have been constructed with only a handful of transistors and switches have displayed convincing animal-like behavior.

The beginnings of a brain
As animals developed more sophisticated abilities to move and sense, their nervous systems developed more spatial organization. The nervous system of one type of flatworm is shown below. The animal's sensory organs – two rudimentary eyes and receptors for food – are positioned in front. These nerve cell clusters assumed greater importance and ultimately developed into a rudimentary brain.

Eyes

Food receptors

Rudimentary brain

Longitudinal nerve cords

Nerve twigs to muscles

Patterns of movement
Much of the worm's nerve network forms two nerve cords, from which twigs of nerve fibers branch into muscles in the sides of the worm. The worm's behavior is still based almost entirely on reflex action. Favorable stimuli automatically elicit muscle contractions that move the worm toward the stimulus; unfavorable stimuli cause the worm to retreat.

An advanced nervous system
Like other higher mammals, humans have several highly developed sensory systems (including vision and hearing) and a musculoskeletal system that allows an extensive range of movements. The human nervous system has parts that fulfill functions similar to those in other animals for sensing, coordinating movements, and controlling internal functions. But the most striking feature of the human nervous system is the huge cerebrum, largely devoted to activities unique to humans, such as sophisticated memory and learning ability, language, problem-solving, and creative thought.

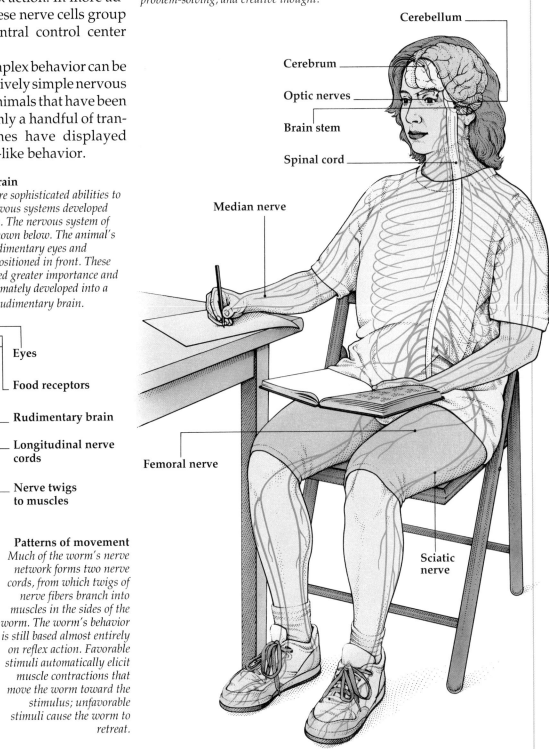

Cerebellum

Cerebrum

Optic nerves

Brain stem

Spinal cord

Median nerve

Femoral nerve

Sciatic nerve

EVOLUTION AND DEVELOPMENT

As the human brain grows in the embryo, it passes through a series of stages. These stages correspond to the evolution of the brain in lower animals. The human brain first resembles an amphibian's brain, then a reptile's, then a bird's. In short, the human brain's embryonic development parallels its own evolution.

DEVELOPMENT OF THE EMBRYO

The brain and nervous system are among the first body parts to specialize and function in the embryo. Most changes occur in the first few weeks of life. All nerve cells have been formed by the time of birth.

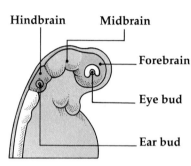

At 3 weeks
During early embryonic development, a tube appears along the back of the embryo. This is the neural tube, from which the entire nervous system develops. At the top of the tube, three bulges develop to form the three main divisions of the brain – the forebrain, the midbrain, and the hindbrain. Eye and ear buds also emerge by the end of the third week. The lower part of the neural tube is the forerunner of the spinal cord.

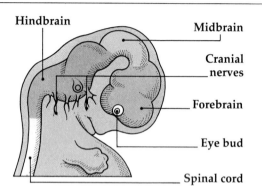

At 7 weeks
The parts of the developing neural tube initially form a straight line, but the tube soon bends so that the forebrain and hindbrain are at right angles to each other. The hindbrain develops rapidly at this stage and begins to sprout a series of nerves (cranial nerves). The forebrain also begins to enlarge, forming two bulges. These will become the large, folded cerebrum and underlying structures, such as the thalamus.

HOW DO OUR BRAINS COMPARE WITH ANIMAL BRAINS?

As animals move up the evolutionary chain, their hindbrains become more complex. Their forebrains progressively enlarge, reaching maximum size in humans.

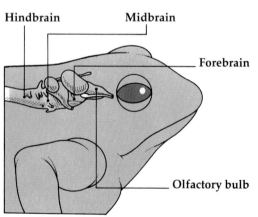

Amphibian brain
The brain of an adult frog shows roughly the same level of development as that of a 3-week-old human embryo. Although its hindbrain is moderately developed, the frog's forebrain is small, and one of its largest parts (the olfactory bulb) at the front governs only the sense of smell.

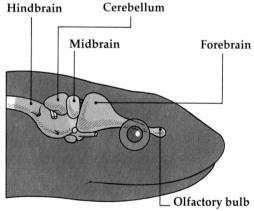

Reptile brain
The brain of an adult reptile corresponds to that of a 7-week-old human embryo. The reptile brain lacks forebrain development, although both hindbrain and forebrain are more developed than the amphibian's, to accommodate the superior abilities of a land-based animal. There is still a large olfactory area.

Spot the difference?
The human embryo at 5 weeks can hardly be differentiated from the embryo of a reptile, bird, or rabbit. They all have similar nervous systems with primitive brains in the form of small bulges at the head of the neural tube.

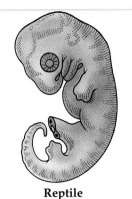
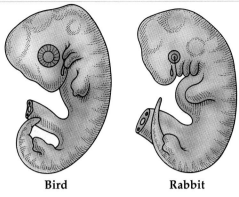
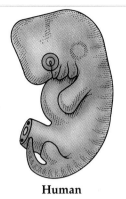

Reptile   **Bird**   **Rabbit**   **Human**

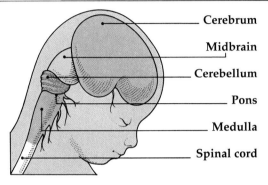

Cerebrum
Midbrain
Cerebellum
Pons
Medulla
Spinal cord

At 11 weeks
By this stage, most features of the adult brain appear in rudimentary form. The hindbrain differentiates into the cerebellum (largely concerned with balance and coordination) and the pons and medulla (which control vital functions such as breathing and heartbeat). Meanwhile, the forebrain continues to grow, and the bulk of it – the cerebrum – begins to overlap the underlying structures.

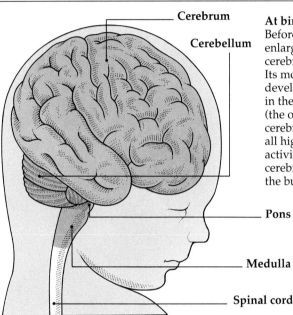

Cerebrum
Cerebellum
Pons
Medulla
Spinal cord

At birth
Before birth, massive enlargement of the cerebrum continues. Its most impressive development occurs in the cerebral cortex (the outer layers of the cerebrum) – the site of all higher conscious activity. At birth, the cerebrum makes up the bulk of the brain.

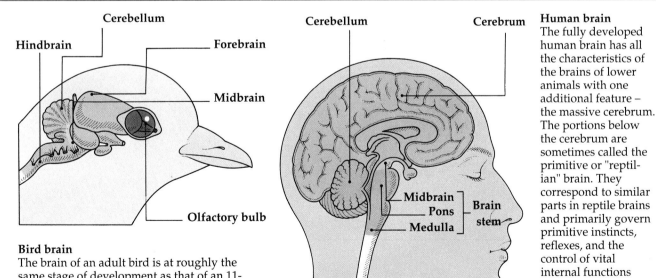

Cerebellum
Hindbrain
Forebrain
Midbrain
Olfactory bulb

Cerebellum
Cerebrum
Midbrain
Pons
Medulla
Brain stem
Spinal cord

Bird brain
The brain of an adult bird is at roughly the same stage of development as that of an 11-week-old human embryo. The bird's cerebellum is comparatively large, to achieve the balance and motor coordination required for flight. The forebrain is also enlarged but is still tiny compared with the human forebrain.

Human brain
The fully developed human brain has all the characteristics of the brains of lower animals with one additional feature – the massive cerebrum. The portions below the cerebrum are sometimes called the primitive or "reptilian" brain. They correspond to similar parts in reptile brains and primarily govern primitive instincts, reflexes, and the control of vital internal functions such as breathing and heartbeat.

HOW IS THE NERVOUS SYSTEM ORGANIZED?

The brain/computer analogy
Many similarities exist between your brain and a computer: they have similar types of inputs and outputs, have large data-storage (memory) systems, and can call up a variety of operating programs to perform specific functions and skills. While most computer programs can only be improved externally, your brain can constantly update many of its own programs to perfect such skills as playing golf or knitting a sweater.

The human nervous system has two parts – the central nervous system and the peripheral nervous system.

Central nervous system

Your central nervous system consists of your brain and your spinal cord. They act as your body's central coordinating and processing unit.

Peripheral nervous system

The nerves that emanate from the central nervous system to all parts of your body make up your peripheral nervous system. This system includes all five of your senses. The peripheral nervous system also has two parts: a somatic system and an autonomic system. The somatic system gathers information about the outside world, transmits it to the central nervous system, and sends signals from there to your body's skeletal muscles, causing them to move.

The autonomic system regulates your body's internal environment. It carries information from inside the body to the central nervous system and transmits the information to organs, such as the heart, which work automatically. The autonomic system is divided into the sympathetic and parasympathetic systems (see page 70).

Nerve cells

Cells that send signals are called nerve cells, or neurons (see page 16). Each has a cell body and at least one long extension (axon) that carries the signal to its target. Nerves contain thousands of individual nerve cell fibers.

IS THE BRAIN LIKE A COMPUTER?

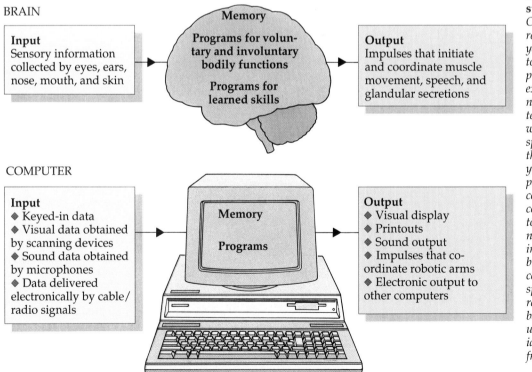

BRAIN

Input
Sensory information collected by eyes, ears, nose, mouth, and skin

Memory
Programs for voluntary and involuntary bodily functions

Programs for learned skills

Output
Impulses that initiate and coordinate muscle movement, speech, and glandular secretions

COMPUTER

Input
◆ Keyed-in data
◆ Visual data obtained by scanning devices
◆ Sound data obtained by microphones
◆ Data delivered electronically by cable/radio signals

Memory

Programs

Output
◆ Visual display
◆ Printouts
◆ Sound output
◆ Impulses that coordinate robotic arms
◆ Electronic output to other computers

Brains and supercomputers
One of the most remarkable aspects of your brain is its ability to "run" several programs at once. For example, it can simultaneously control body temperature, coordinate walking movements and speech, and engage in thought. To approach your brain's level of performance, separate computers or sections of computers would have to be operated simultaneously, with numerous interconnections. Your brain also outperforms a computer at certain specific skills, such as recognizing connections between apparently unconnected ideas and identifying whole objects from only a small part.

CENTRAL NERVOUS SYSTEM

The central nervous system consists of the brain and spinal cord. It is entirely encased in bone – the brain inside the skull and the spinal cord inside the backbone, or spinal column.

Brain

Your brain is the control center of your body. It receives a constant barrage of sensory information about the environment and your body's inner functioning. It processes this information, compares it with stored data, and decides whether action is needed to adapt to the environment or to adjust some internal bodily function. The brain also serves as the body's storehouse for data and is the seat of consciousness and emotion.

Spinal cord

Your spinal cord can process and initiate responses to many types of sensory information at an unconscious, automatic level. It also consists of bundles – or tracts – of nerve fibers that transmit information between your brain and other parts of your body.

Lumbar plexus

Sacral plexus

PERIPHERAL NERVOUS SYSTEM

The peripheral nervous system provides the "cabling" that connects the central nervous system to its input sites (sensory organs and receptors) and output devices (muscles and glands).

Cranial nerves

These 12 pairs of nerves connect directly to the brain. Some transmit information from sensory organs such as your eyes or nose, some relay motor information to muscles or glands, and some have mixed motor and sensory functions.

Sensory receptors

(not shown)
Sensory receptors reside not only in your eyes, ears, nose, taste buds, and skin but also in your internal organs. Internal receptors include those that collect information about the internal state of the body, including blood pressure and the state of contraction of each muscle.

Brachial plexus

Spinal nerves

The 31 pairs of spinal nerves emerge from the spinal cord and supply all parts of your trunk and limbs. Each of the spinal nerves contains both sensory and motor fibers. In the upper chest and lower abdomen, the nerves join to form concentrated networks called plexuses that serve the limbs.

Sympathetic nerve trunks

Chains of ganglia (clusters of nerve cells) form part of the sympathetic division of your autonomic nervous system. They act as relay stations for information passing from your central nervous system to body organs such as the salivary glands, heart, lungs, and digestive organs.

15

NERVE CELLS

Nerve cells are the remarkable building blocks of the nervous system. They are also known as neurons. Neurons receive, analyze, coordinate, and transmit information inside your body. There are approximately 100,000,000,000 neurons in the human brain. Extraordinary as this number is, even more extraordinary is the fact that in a healthy person each of these individual cells works harmoniously and almost instantaneously with all the others to generate normal functioning of your organs, senses, muscles, and thoughts.

NERVE CELL STRUCTURE

Like other cells of the body, nerve cells possess a membrane that encloses cytoplasm and a nucleus. But nerve cells have become extremely specialized so they can transfer information. Their shape and biochemical properties reflect this function. The characteristics of a typical nerve cell are illustrated here.

Axon
This long, thin extension of the nerve cell membrane contains cytoplasm and arises from a thickened area of the cell body known as the axon hillock. The axon carries information away from the cell body to an appropriate target, such as a muscle, a gland, or another nerve cell. Axons can range in length from a few millimeters to 6 feet or more, and most terminate at a small number of targets. For example, a single motor nerve cell transmits information to a relatively small number of muscle fibers. But some axons within the brain make many more connections.

Nodes of Ranvier
These spaces occur between the bundles of glial cells that form the myelin sheath.

Terminal fibers
At its end, the axon divides into thin branches called axon terminal fibers, which are covered with tiny enlargements called synaptic knobs.

Myelin sheath
The axons of certain types of nerve cells are covered with a fatty substance known as myelin, formed from glial cells, the other group of cells in the nervous system. A coating of myelin permits faster transmission of nerve impulses by insulating the axon.

Synaptic knobs
These tiny protuberances release a chemical compound called a neurotransmitter that moves across the minute gap (synapse) between one nerve cell and another. This process triggers an electrical signal in an adjoining nerve cell.

A nerve cell under the microscope
A scanning electron microscope produced this color-enhanced image of a nerve cell from the brain. The yellow nerve cell has a triangular cell body extending into a single axon (at top left), which divides into several fibers. The other two extensions of the cell body are dendrites.

Cell body
The main body of the cell, also called the soma, contains the cell nucleus and materials for its maintenance and functioning. The shape and size of the cell body vary among different types of neurons.

Nucleus

Axon hillock

Dendrites
These branchlike extensions that originate from the cell body are named from the Greek word "dendron," meaning tree. Dendrites receive information from connecting nerve endings via a neurotransmitter, convert the chemical signal into an electrical impulse, and conduct this impulse toward the cell body. Each dendrite has enough surface area to support many synapses, enabling the cell to receive input from thousands of other nerve cells.

GLIAL CELLS

Nerve cells account for only 5 to 10 percent of all cells in the nervous system. Far more numerous is a second group of cells, known as glial cells, which cannot transmit information. Instead, glial cells provide protection, nutrition, and structural support for nerve cells. Several types of glial cells (examples shown below) occur in both the central nervous system and the peripheral nervous system. Some glial cells produce proteins, called neurotrophic factors, that stimulate the growth of nerve cells during normal development and after injury. Researchers are attempting to find out whether these proteins could be used to prevent degeneration of injured nerve cells in disorders such as Parkinson's disease and Alzheimer's disease.

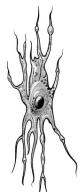

An oligodendroglial cell
This type of glial cell forms the myelin sheath that surrounds the large axons of nerve cells in the central nervous system. Schwann cells perform the same function in the peripheral nervous system.

An astrocyte
Astrocytes (along with ependymal cells) help form the blood-brain barrier, which controls the entry of substances, including medications, into the brain via the bloodstream. Astrocytes and other glial cells known as microglia also help form scar tissue after injury.

NERVE CELL BEHAVIOR

Just as the most complex computer contains a vast number of simple on/off switches, your body contains a multitude of individual nerve cells, each responding to stimuli by transmitting a single nerve impulse. Triggered by a stimulus, the nerve cell generates a nerve impulse – a zone of electrical charge – that moves along the surface of the cell. This signal travels down the cell body's extension, known as the axon, and releases a chemical (neurotransmitter) from the terminals at the axon's end. This chemical may stimulate a second nerve cell to generate an electrical signal. In this way, a message is carried through the pathway of interconnected nerve cells (called a neural arc) to distant parts of the body where the response occurs.

Nerve cells obey an all-or-nothing law. If a stimulus is strong enough, the cell will transmit its electrical signal along its axon. If a stimulus is not strong enough, nothing happens. This may seem strange since we can tell the difference between the pain of a minor cut on the hand and the throb of a severe toothache. But the sensation's intensity does not depend on the strength of the nerve cell's response. It depends on the number of nerve cells that are stimulated and on their frequency of response. A strong stimulus makes a nerve cell "fire" more often.

HOW DO NERVE CELLS COMMUNICATE?

Your nerve cells communicate with each other and with your muscles or glands. This communication proceeds during the series of events described below. All of these complex processes occur within a fraction of a second.

2 When the nerve cell becomes stimulated, channels in its outer membrane temporarily open to ions (atoms with an electrical charge) in the surrounding fluid. Positively charged ions, such as sodium and potassium, then rush through the channels, giving the inside of the cell membrane a local positive charge.

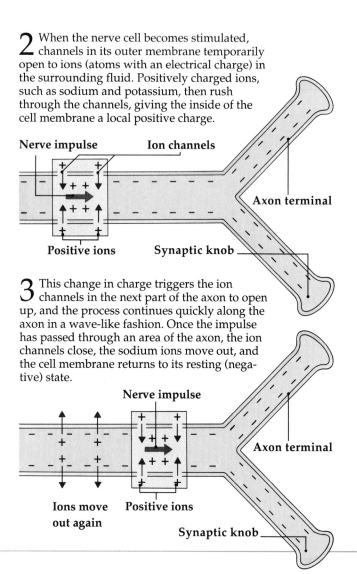

3 This change in charge triggers the ion channels in the next part of the axon to open up, and the process continues quickly along the axon in a wave-like fashion. Once the impulse has passed through an area of the axon, the ion channels close, the sodium ions move out, and the cell membrane returns to its resting (negative) state.

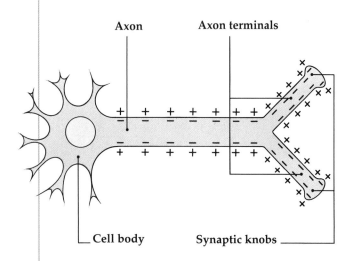

1 When a nerve cell is not transmitting or receiving a message, it is in a resting state. During this state, the inside of the nerve cell membrane has a negative electrical charge because the cell constantly emits sodium ions, which are positive.

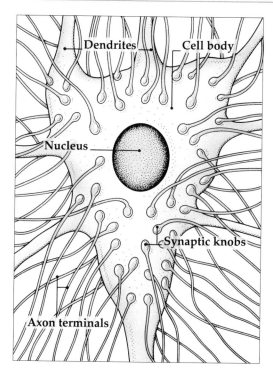

Dendrites
Cell body
Nucleus
Synaptic knobs
Axon terminals

Each nerve cell transmits information to only a small number of recipients. But it can receive input from many other nerve cells. The speed with which an axon conducts an impulse depends on its size and other properties. Small axons can conduct impulses at a velocity of only around 1.5 feet per second. Large axons can transmit impulses to their target nerve cells at a speed of approximately 400 feet per second. Many nerve cell axons have an insulating cover – the myelin sheath – that increases the speed of nerve impulse transmission.

A cell body covered with synaptic knobs

The surface area of a nerve cell is large enough to receive information from many other nerve cells via tiny synaptic knobs that connect with the cell body and its dendrites, as shown at left.

CAN NERVE CELLS BE REPLACED?

Nerve cells do not divide, and the cells from which they originate are absent in adults. This means that the death of a nerve cell represents a permanent loss. Damage to the nervous system may be irreversible. But damaged nerve fibers (axons) in parts of the body other than the brain or spinal cord can grow again and reestablish connections with their targets. Undamaged nerve cells near an injury site can also establish new connections to partially restore function. With the expanded use of alternate nerve cell pathways, this regrowth plays an important role in the rehabilitation of patients after nervous system injury or illness, such as a stroke, or after neurosurgery.

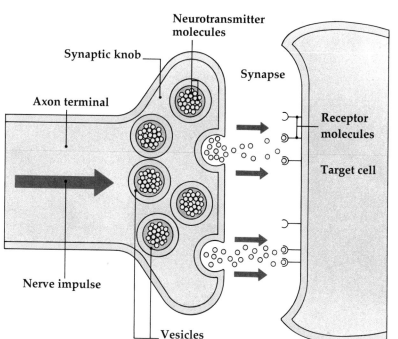

Neurotransmitter molecules
Synaptic knob
Synapse
Axon terminal
Receptor molecules
Target cell
Nerve impulse
Vesicles

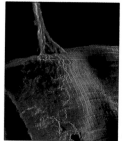

A neuromuscular junction

Above, a motor neuron (pink) ends on the surface of a skeletal muscle cell (magnified 300 times).

4 Electrical impulses reach the axon terminals and trigger the release of a neurotransmitter, contained in small spheres called vesicles. The vesicles, which are bound to the surface of the synaptic knob, spill their contents into the gap, or synapse, between the synaptic knob and the target cell's surface. Once across the gap, the neurotransmitter molecules bind to specific receptor molecules on the target cell's surface and activate a response. For example, if the target is a muscle cell, the effect might be contraction of the muscle fiber.

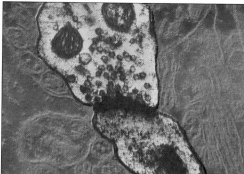

A synapse between two nerve cells

This color-enhanced photograph (magnified 34,200 times) shows a synapse (gap) between two nerve cells (yellow) in the cerebral cortex. The synaptic gap appears as a deep red strip, and the vesicles that contain neurotransmitters appear as red/yellow spheres.

THE BRAIN

The living brain is a soft, easily compressible mass of grayish white tissue with a heavily folded surface. Bright red arteries and purple veins course through this grooved mass. The brain and its blood vessels lie completely enclosed inside three layers of membranes, called the meninges. The outer layer forms a tough, protective coat. The brain weighs about 3 pounds and contains a tremendous number of nerve cells and supporting glial cells.

The cerebrum
The illustration above shows where the brain lies in the skull. The largest part of the human brain is the cerebrum, which consists of two cerebral hemispheres.

Cerebrum

STRUCTURE OF THE BRAIN

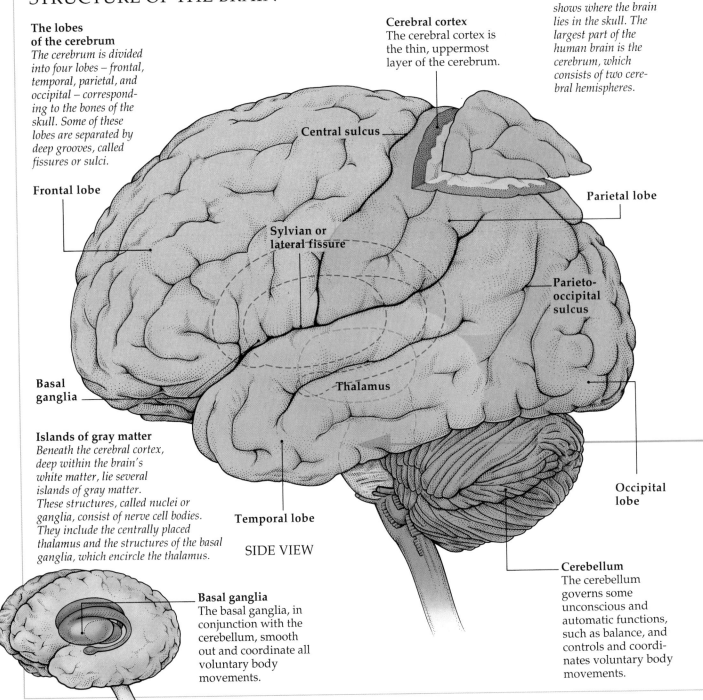

The lobes of the cerebrum
The cerebrum is divided into four lobes – frontal, temporal, parietal, and occipital – corresponding to the bones of the skull. Some of these lobes are separated by deep grooves, called fissures or sulci.

Cerebral cortex
The cerebral cortex is the thin, uppermost layer of the cerebrum.

Central sulcus

Frontal lobe

Sylvian or lateral fissure

Parietal lobe

Parieto-occipital sulcus

Basal ganglia

Thalamus

Islands of gray matter
Beneath the cerebral cortex, deep within the brain's white matter, lie several islands of gray matter. These structures, called nuclei or ganglia, consist of nerve cell bodies. They include the centrally placed thalamus and the structures of the basal ganglia, which encircle the thalamus.

Temporal lobe

SIDE VIEW

Occipital lobe

Cerebellum
The cerebellum governs some unconscious and automatic functions, such as balance, and controls and coordinates voluntary body movements.

Basal ganglia
The basal ganglia, in conjunction with the cerebellum, smooth out and coordinate all voluntary body movements.

The longitudinal fissure

The two hemispheres

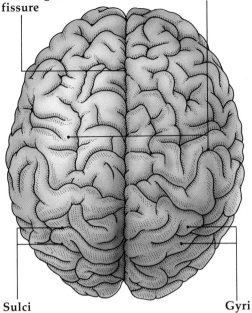

Sulci

Gyri

TOP VIEW

Gyri and sulci

The surface of the cerebrum is heavily folded, forming numerous ridges and deep clefts. A raised area is called a gyrus and a single groove is known as a sulcus. Some of the larger sulci are called fissures.

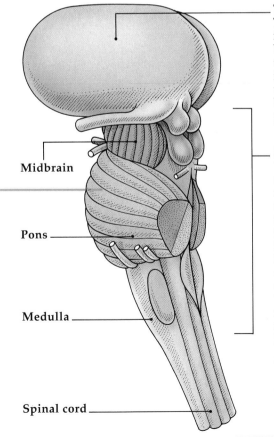

Midbrain

Pons

Medulla

Spinal cord

Corpus callosum
The two halves of the brain are connected by the corpus callosum, a massive communication trunk that contains more than 200 million nerve fibers. Surprisingly, cutting the corpus callosum has little effect on personality, intellect, or other brain functions.

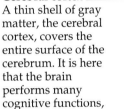

Cerebral cortex
A thin shell of gray matter, the cerebral cortex, covers the entire surface of the cerebrum. It is here that the brain performs many cognitive functions, such as thinking and remembering. Numerous infoldings of the cortex allow its large surface area to fit inside the skull.

Thalamus
The thalamus relays information about bodily sensations to the cortex and sends information about what is going on in the body to many other parts of the brain.

Brain stem
The brain stem, composed of the midbrain, pons, and medulla, contains the tracts of nerve fibers that connect the brain to the rest of the body by way of the spinal cord. The brain stem contains the nerve cell bodies for some of the nerves that supply the face and head. It also houses centers responsible for breathing, heart rate, and controlling the levels of wakeful consciousness and sleep.

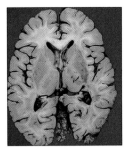

Gray and white matter
Parts of the brain are gray, others are white. Gray matter consists of nerve cell bodies. White matter is composed of nerve fibers that connect the brain and nervous system.

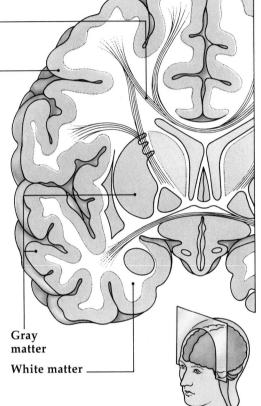

Gray matter

White matter

DIVISIONS OF THE BRAIN

For descriptive purposes, the parts of the brain are often divided as follows:

FOREBRAIN
◆ **Cerebrum**
   Cortex
   Basal ganglia
◆ **Diencephalon**
   Thalamus
   Hypothalamus

MIDBRAIN
HINDBRAIN   ⎫
◆ **Pons**   ⎬ BRAIN STEM
◆ **Medulla**   ⎭
◆ **Cerebellum**

PROTECTION AND NOURISHMENT

For protection, the soft, vulnerable tissues of the brain and spinal cord are encased in bone and wrapped in three layers of membranes, called the meninges. Further protection is provided by cerebrospinal fluid, which cushions the brain and spinal cord during movement.

Cerebrospinal fluid is a clear, watery liquid similar in chemical composition to the fluid in which blood cells are suspended. Cerebrospinal fluid is produced inside the ventricles (cavities) of the brain and surrounds the brain and spinal cord, both of which actually float in this liquid. Its main function is to provide protection against injury. Cerebrospinal fluid contains glucose (sugar), proteins, and electrolytes (conductors of electrical charges), such as sodium and chlorides. When doctors suspect a person has inflammation of the central nervous system, they measure the concentrations of these elements in the fluid through a procedure called lumbar puncture (see page 105).

**Protective coverings
of the brain and spinal cord**
Three layers of membranes, called the meninges, protect the brain and spinal cord. The inner layer – the pia mater – adheres to the surface of the brain and spinal cord. The middle layer – the arachnoid – forms a web that extends to the pia mater. The subarachnoid space, between the arachnoid and the pia mater, contains cerebrospinal fluid. The outermost layer – the tough, fibrous dura mater – binds tightly to the inside of the skull but only loosely to the vertebral canal.

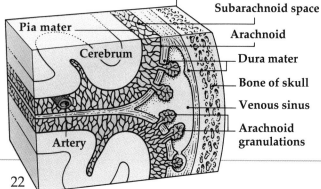

Subarachnoid space
Pia mater
Cerebrum
Arachnoid
Dura mater
Bone of skull
Venous sinus
Arachnoid granulations
Artery

The ventricles of the brain
The brain contains four interconnecting cavities (ventricles). The two lateral ventricles, also called the first and second ventricles, and the third ventricle are located in the cerebrum; the fourth ventricle lies in the brain stem. Each lateral ventricle connects to the third ventricle via a hole called the interventricular foramen.

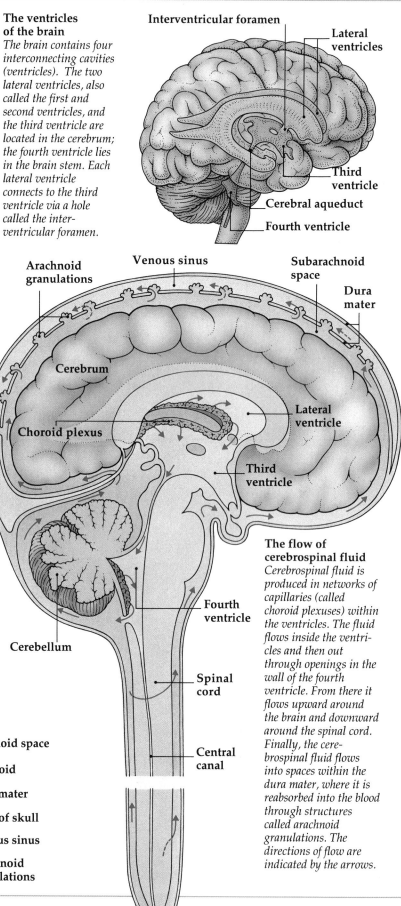

Interventricular foramen
Lateral ventricles
Third ventricle
Cerebral aqueduct
Fourth ventricle

Arachnoid granulations
Venous sinus
Subarachnoid space
Dura mater
Cerebrum
Choroid plexus
Lateral ventricle
Third ventricle
Cerebellum
Fourth ventricle
Spinal cord
Central canal

The flow of cerebrospinal fluid
Cerebrospinal fluid is produced in networks of capillaries (called choroid plexuses) within the ventricles. The fluid flows inside the ventricles and then out through openings in the wall of the fourth ventricle. From there it flows upward around the brain and downward around the spinal cord. Finally, the cerebrospinal fluid flows into spaces within the dura mater, where it is reabsorbed into the blood through structures called arachnoid granulations. The directions of flow are indicated by the arrows.

Blood supply to the brain

The brain quickly loses its ability to function without a continuous supply of oxygen, glucose (sugar), and other nutrients, which are provided via the bloodstream. It needs an enormous supply of blood for its size: 20 percent of the body's blood supply is channeled to the brain at all times.

If blood flow, or the oxygen or glucose that it supplies to the brain, is reduced or completely cut off, irreversible damage can occur very rapidly. Drowning, heart attacks, strokes, and even severe asthmatic attacks can damage the brain by disrupting the supply of one or more of these vital elements. If the blood supply is terminated at normal temperatures for more than about 4 to 8 minutes, a vegetative state or death is inevitable.

The blood-brain barrier

Glucose and other substances needed by the brain pass to it from the blood circulating inside the capillaries (small blood vessels). But a special structure called the blood-brain barrier controls the passage of many substances into the brain. The blood-brain barrier protects the brain against some infectious agents, but it also complicates the treatment of brain infections. Most antibiotics, including penicillin, do not cross this barrier, nor do drugs used to treat cancer.

To make certain that medications pass across the blood-brain barrier, doctors sometimes inject them directly into the cerebrospinal fluid. In other cases, the molecular structure of a drug is redesigned. For example, symptoms of Parkinson's disease are caused by a lack of the chemical dopamine in the brain. Although dopamine cannot cross the blood-brain barrier, the drug levodopa is able to cross in small quantities and is converted into dopamine in the brain. A third, more experimental treatment alters the composition of the bloodstream in a way that causes a temporary opening of the blood-brain barrier.

Blood supply to the brain
Four major arteries supply blood to the brain: two large carotid arteries that run up both sides of the front of the neck and two vertebral arteries that pass up through holes in the bones at the back of the neck. The carotid arteries divide into internal and external branches. The external carotid arteries supply the face and the surface of the head. The internal carotid arteries and the vertebral arteries end at a circle at the base of the brain called the circle of Willis. From there, major branches arise and supply the brain itself by way of smaller branches.

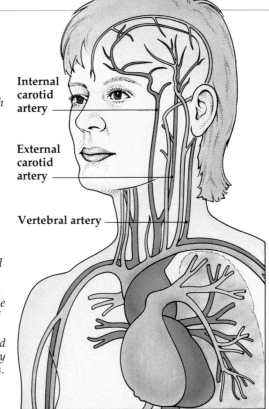

Internal carotid artery

External carotid artery

Vertebral artery

Network of arteries in the brain
This color-enhanced X-ray, obtained after the injection of a dye through which X-rays cannot pass, shows the extensive arterial network that supplies the brain.

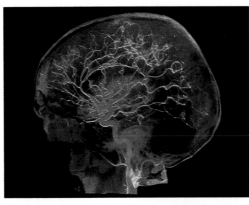

Structure of the blood-brain barrier
The blood-brain barrier consists of two layers, which prevent the entry of many types of molecules into the brain. The first layer is made up of endothelial cells lining the capillaries that supply the brain. These cells are impermeable. The cells also form a biochemical barrier by rejecting certain substances. The second layer consists of glial cells, whose fibers encase the capillaries, as an additional barrier.

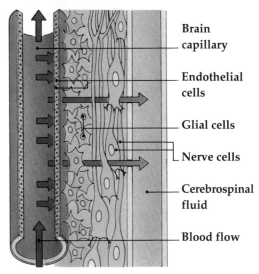

Brain capillary

Endothelial cells

Glial cells

Nerve cells

Cerebrospinal fluid

Blood flow

THE HUMAN CEREBRAL CORTEX

Brain researchers have mapped much of the cerebral cortex into areas that serve known functions. We can now pinpoint accurately the sites of the cortex concerned with voluntary movement, bodily sensations (such as touch, pain, and temperature), hearing, vision, smell, taste, and the processing and interpretation of incoming information. The cerebral cortex is also the seat of all higher human functions, such as intellect, memory, talent, and emotion.

Areas of cortex adjacent to sites of known function are called association areas. These areas occupy more than three fourths of the cortex. The association areas interpret the various types of information (such as touch and vision) received by primary areas in the cortex and translate these stimuli into voluntary and involuntary motor responses. Association areas also regulate the complex processes that underlie higher mental functions, such as memory.

HOW DOES THE CORTEX FUNCTION?

The workings of different areas of the cerebral cortex were initially investigated in two ways. First, researchers observed the effect of damage to, or removal of, parts of the brain. Second, they noted the effects of direct stimulation of the brain by electrodes. Today, doctors use imaging techniques such as positron emission tomography (PET) scanning to "map" brain activity while the subject thinks, looks, listens, speaks, writes, or sings.

THE BRAIN MAP

Prefrontal cortex (thought elaboration)
The prefrontal cortex gives you the ability to concentrate for long periods, to plan for the future, to think through problems, and to modify behavior.

Premotor cortex
The premotor cortex coordinates complex, skilled movements or sequences of movement, such as playing the piano.

Motor cortex
The motor cortex sends instructions to specific sets of muscles causing voluntary movements, such as lifting a fork to your mouth.

Primary somatic sensory cortex
This area receives information directly from the sensory receptors in the skin and can distinguish the specific type of sensation (such as pressure) felt in any region of the body.

Gustatory area (taste)

Somatic sensory association cortex

Visual association cortex

Broca's area (speech)
Broca's area controls speech. It is located in the left hemisphere in almost all right-handed and most left-handed people.

Auditory association cortex

The association areas
The association areas of the cortex further interpret information received by the primary areas. For example, while your primary auditory cortex detects simple qualities of sounds, such as pitch and volume, the auditory association cortex analyzes this information so that you can recognize whole sounds, such as spoken words or musical melodies.

Wernicke's area (general interpretation)
Wernicke's area, which controls the interpretation of the many types of sensory information that enter your brain, is usually well developed in only one (the dominant) hemisphere.

Primary auditory cortex
This area detects the qualities of sounds, such as specific tones, and degrees of loudness.

Primary visual cortex
The primary visual cortex detects relatively simple aspects of the visual scene, such as light and dark, and lines and borders.

"Reading" your bumps

In the early 19th century, before scientists understood the brain as we do today, phrenology – "reading" the bumps on a person's skull – enjoyed great popularity. Phrenologists claimed that by feeling or measuring the skull they could evaluate a person's personality and capabilities. All human faculties were said to be precisely localized in the brain, with enlarged areas of the skull indicating the locations of the most highly developed faculties. The idea has no scientific basis.

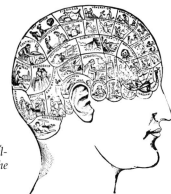

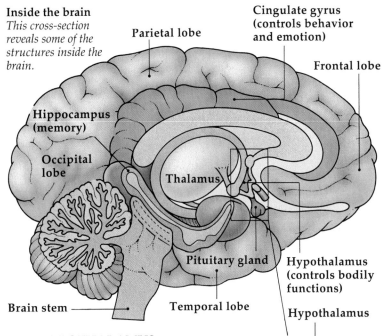

The nerve cells of the cortex

A thin, stained section of the cerebral cortex (magnified 60 times) reveals different shapes and sizes of nerve cells and their threadlike connecting fibers. Some nerve cells primarily send electrical impulses to other parts of the nervous system. The principal job of other cells is to receive incoming information. The percentages of different types of nerve cells vary from one area of the cortex to another, depending on that area's function.

THE PRIMITIVE BRAIN

The limbic system is the part of the brain that governs subconscious instincts and emotions. Many experts regard it as primitive because its functions appeared early in the evolution of the brain. The limbic system links higher brain centers, used to think or remember, with lower structures that coordinate automatic bodily functions, such as breathing. The limbic system encircles the top of the brain stem. It consists of hidden areas of cortex and deeper brain structures. The areas of the limbic cortex sit on the inner sides of the cerebral hemispheres around the corpus callosum. An important part of the limbic cortex is the arch-shaped cingulate gyrus, which lies directly above the corpus callosum. The cingulate gyrus controls emotional responses, such as rage and fright.

Continuous with this same ring of cortex is the hippocampus, lying along the inner border of the temporal lobe. The hippocampus and related structures are involved in memory storage.

The structures and functions of the limbic system are covered in more detail in Chapter 3 on page 74.

SENSE OF SMELL

The sense of smell is perceived by parts of your limbic system, called olfactory areas, that are located on the inner surface of each hemisphere. The close links between the olfactory areas and other structures of your limbic system help explain why your sense of smell can make you recall strong, emotionally charged memories.

Inside the brain

This cross-section reveals some of the structures inside the brain.

Parietal lobe

Cingulate gyrus (controls behavior and emotion)

Frontal lobe

Hippocampus (memory)

Occipital lobe

Thalamus

Pituitary gland

Hypothalamus (controls bodily functions)

Hypothalamus

Brain stem

Temporal lobe

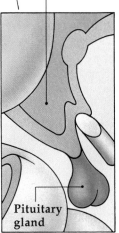

Pituitary gland

THE HYPOTHALAMUS

Just below the thalamus, near the middle of the base of the brain, lies the hypothalamus. This tiny structure's workings are linked with those of the limbic system. The hypothalamus is the site at which the nervous and hormonal systems interact. Brain signals, including those associated with thought and emotion, cause the hypothalamus to send chemicals to the pituitary gland. These chemicals adjust the release of hormones that regulate bodily functions. The hypothalamus is discussed in more detail in Chapter 3 on page 69.

BRAIN CHEMICALS

Nerve cells communicate through chemicals called neurotransmitters (see NERVE CELL BEHAVIOR on page 18). Some neurotransmitters are inhibitory, which means that they cause nerve cells to become less easily activated. Other neurotransmitters are excitatory, which means that they cause other nerve cells to be more easily activated. Many different types of neurotransmitters have been discovered in the brain, and research into their functions continues.

One important neurotransmitter that has an inhibitory effect on other nerve cells is called gamma-aminobutyric acid (GABA). GABA reduces anxiety. Antianxiety drugs, such as diazepam, enhance the effects of GABA in the brain. Loss of inhibitory GABA nerve terminals in the cortex may cause increased excitability of nerve cells in people with epilepsy, resulting in seizures.

Glutamate, a neurotransmitter that has an excitatory effect, helps to form long-term memories. The neurotransmitter dopamine has several significant functions. Loss of dopamine-containing nerve

Cerebral cortex

Corpus callosum

Nucleus basalis of Meynert

Acetylcholine containing nerve fiber

A chemical that affects higher mental functions

Acetylcholine is a neurotransmitter that seems to direct and maintain attention. Higher intellectual functions, such as learning and memory, require controlled attention. A large cluster of nerve cells containing this neurotransmitter resides in a structure near the base of the forebrain called the nucleus basalis of Meynert. These nerve cells send nerve fibers to vast areas of the cerebral cortex, where the acetylcholine is released and has its effects. In Alzheimer's disease, characterized by increasing loss of mental function (dementia), a severe loss of acetylcholine-containing cells is evident in the nucleus basalis of Meynert and adjacent areas.

THE BRAIN'S NATURAL OPIATES

In the 1970s, scientists discovered brain receptor sites that responded to opiate drugs, such as morphine. Researchers also found that molecules similar to morphine were produced in the brain. They named these substances endorphins (endogenous morphinelike substances). Released during vigorous exercise, endorphins help relieve pain. This explains why athletes injured during a game can continue playing without pain. Endorphins also help control responses to stress and can improve mood, explaining the sense of well-being athletes report after working out.

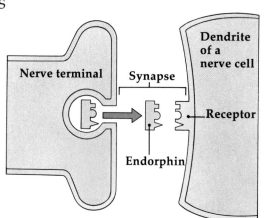

Nerve terminal

Synapse

Dendrite of a nerve cell

Receptor

Endorphin

What are endorphins?

An endorphin is a type of neurotransmitter released by specific endorphin-containing nerve terminals. It attaches to a receptor on another nerve cell, like a key that fits a lock, to influence the nerve cell's activity.

DRUGS USED TO TREAT BRAIN DISORDERS

Doctors think some brain disorders are caused by deficiencies of neurotransmitters in the brain. Researchers are attempting to develop drugs that will replace or replenish the neurotransmitters or mimic their effects. For disorders caused by too much of a particular neurochemical, researchers are developing drugs to block the effects of the natural chemical at its receptor.

cells in one area of the brain characterizes the movement disorder known as Parkinson's disease (see page 116). Some inconclusive research studies suggest that overactivity of dopamine-containing cells in another region of the brain may cause schizophrenia.

Norepinephrine is a modulatory neurotransmitter that selectively enhances or reduces the effects of other neurotransmitters. It selects important information for our attention that groups of cells in the brain transmit to other nerve cells. Norepinephrine helps us cope with emergency situations when released outside the brain in response to stimulation by acetylcholine, another neurotransmitter. In some people with depression, brain norepinephrine levels are abnormally low. Certain antidepressant drugs prolong the effects of norepinephrine in the brain.

THE BRAIN AND AGING

Aging is a normal process that occurs at a rate largely determined by genetics. As we age, we progressively lose nerve cells from certain parts of the brain, particularly the cerebral cortex. This cell loss reveals itself in widening of the fissures and narrowing of the elevations on the surface of the brain. Aging brains have been found to lose white matter faster than they lose gray matter.

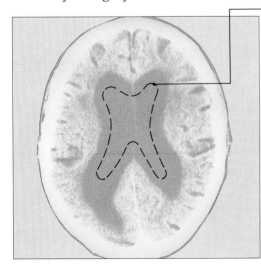

Normal ventricles

Aging and dementia
Changes in the brain's appearance do not necessarily indicate a decline in intellectual performance. But in Alzheimer's disease, marked by dementia, greater than normal loss of cortex occurs in the brain, along with enlargement of the ventricles, as seen on this magnetic resonance imaging (MRI) scan.

NEUROTRANSMITTERS AND AGING

Neurotransmitters in the brain are constantly broken down and replaced by newly manufactured molecules. These ongoing processes tend to become less efficient with age, leading to altered functioning of some neurotransmitter systems. This may help explain how some bodily functions, such as sleep patterns, mood, appetite, hormone function, memory, and motor activity, change as we age.

ASK YOUR DOCTOR
THE BRAIN'S SPECIAL NEEDS

Q **I have insulin-dependent diabetes mellitus. Why has my doctor warned me against overdosing with my insulin?**

A An insulin overdose may cause a low blood glucose level (hypoglycemia). Glucose provides your brain with energy so that it can function properly. Most cases of insulin overdose cause only brief hypoglycemia, resulting in trembling, faintness, rapid heart rate, and, in rare cases, loss of consciousness. In older people, hypoglycemia can be especially dangerous because if the hypoglycemia is prolonged or severe, brain damage can occur. Carry glucose tablets or candy with you to take at the first sign of these symptoms.

Q **My grandfather has been complaining of heart palpitations, and yesterday he fainted. What could be wrong? Should he see his doctor?**

A Too rapid or too slow a heart rate will provide an insufficient flow of blood to your grandfather's brain. He should see his doctor, who will want to determine what type of altered heart rhythm is occurring. His doctor will probably order a test called resting electrocardiography, which measures the heart's rate, rhythm, and form of electrical impulses. Your grandfather may then be asked to wear a Holter monitor, which will record his heart rhythm for a period of 24 hours. The abnormal rhythm can be corrected with medication or by surgical insertion of a pacemaker.

THE SPINAL CORD AND PERIPHERAL NERVES

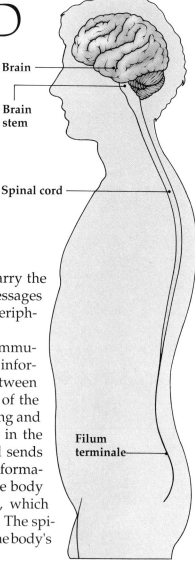

Brain

Brain stem

Spinal cord

Filum terminale

The spinal cord, the lower extension of the brain, forms a critical part of your central nervous system. The peripheral nerves, which consist of the cranial and spinal nerves, connect the brain and spinal cord to all areas of your body. Along with all the sensory and motor receptors of the body, these nerves form the peripheral nervous system.

THE SPINAL CORD

The spinal cord, which extends from the base of your brain, consists of an inner core of gray tissue – the gray matter – surrounded by an outer cylinder of white tissue – the white matter. The gray matter contains nerve cell bodies and nerve cells with short axons (interneurons) and is rich in blood vessels and glial cells. The white matter consists of the axons of nerve cells whose cell bodies may be in the gray matter, in the brain, or outside the central nervous system. These axons, or nerve fibers, extend up to or down from the brain or between different lev-

An elongated extension of the brain
The spinal cord emerges from the skull through a hole called the foramen magnum and forms a column the width of a finger and about 17 inches long. A long strand of membranous tissue, the filum terminale, continues downward from the spinal cord, attaching it to the end of the vertebral column.

els of the spinal cord. They carry the nerve signals that convey messages to and from all parts of the peripheral nervous system.

The spinal cord acts as a communications channel that relays information. Information travels between the brain and different levels of the spinal cord by way of ascending and descending nerve fiber tracts in the white matter. The spinal cord sends information to and receives information from different areas of the body by way of the spinal nerves, which enter and exit the gray matter. The spinal cord also controls many of the body's automatic actions, or reflexes.

THE FIBER TRACTS OF THE WHITE MATTER

The nerve fibers in the white matter transmit information up and down the spinal cord to and from different areas of the brain. All nerve fibers that perform a similar function are grouped together in bundles called fiber tracts.

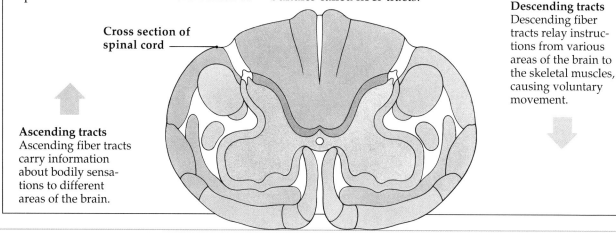

Cross section of spinal cord

Ascending tracts
Ascending fiber tracts carry information about bodily sensations to different areas of the brain.

Descending tracts
Descending fiber tracts relay instructions from various areas of the brain to the skeletal muscles, causing voluntary movement.

STRUCTURE OF THE SPINAL CORD

Protective coverings
Like the brain, the spinal cord is protected by three layers of connective tissue, also called the meninges – the outer dura mater, the middle arachnoid, and the inner pia mater. Cerebrospinal fluid fills the space between the arachnoid and the pia mater.

The vertebral column
The vertebral column, composed of individual bones called vertebrae, houses and protects the spinal cord.

White matter

Gray matter

Nerve fiber tracts

Central canal
Running the length of the spinal cord is a small central canal that contains cerebrospinal fluid.

Pia mater

Arachnoid

Dura mater

Sensory root
Information about bodily sensations runs through sensory nerve fibers and enters the back side of the spinal cord via bundles of fibers known as sensory nerve roots.

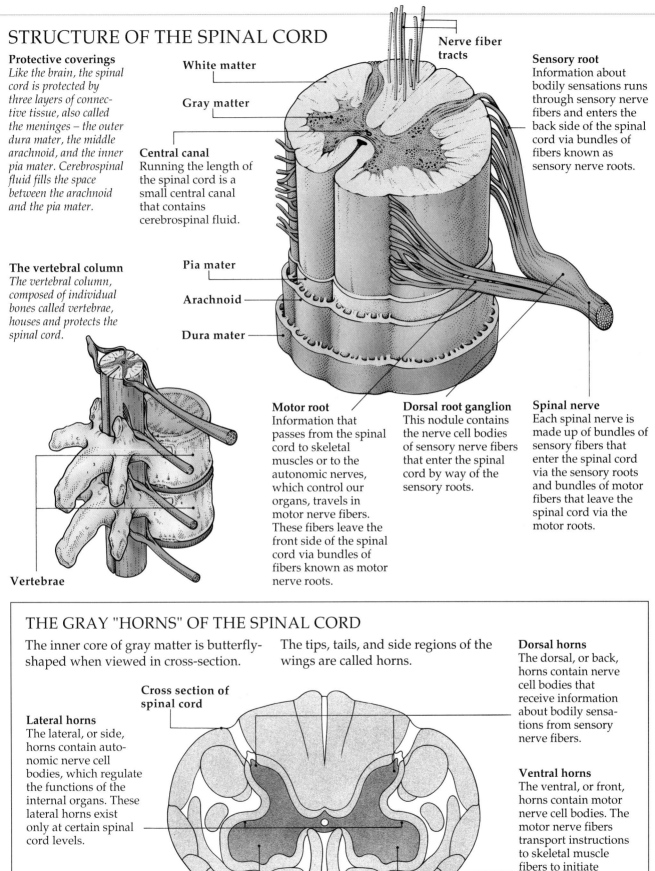

Vertebrae

Motor root
Information that passes from the spinal cord to skeletal muscles or to the autonomic nerves, which control our organs, travels in motor nerve fibers. These fibers leave the front side of the spinal cord via bundles of fibers known as motor nerve roots.

Dorsal root ganglion
This nodule contains the nerve cell bodies of sensory nerve fibers that enter the spinal cord by way of the sensory roots.

Spinal nerve
Each spinal nerve is made up of bundles of sensory fibers that enter the spinal cord via the sensory roots and bundles of motor fibers that leave the spinal cord via the motor roots.

THE GRAY "HORNS" OF THE SPINAL CORD

The inner core of gray matter is butterfly-shaped when viewed in cross-section.

The tips, tails, and side regions of the wings are called horns.

Cross section of spinal cord

Lateral horns
The lateral, or side, horns contain autonomic nerve cell bodies, which regulate the functions of the internal organs. These lateral horns exist only at certain spinal cord levels.

Dorsal horns
The dorsal, or back, horns contain nerve cell bodies that receive information about bodily sensations from sensory nerve fibers.

Ventral horns
The ventral, or front, horns contain motor nerve cell bodies. The motor nerve fibers transport instructions to skeletal muscle fibers to initiate contraction.

THE PERIPHERAL NERVES

Each region of the body is connected to the brain or spinal cord by different types of nerve fibers. Those that receive information about the outside environment and skin sensations from sensory receptors and sensory organs are called somatic sensory fibers. Those nerve fibers that cause skeletal muscles to contract are known as somatic motor nerve fibers. Nerve fibers that regulate internal organ and gland functions are called autonomic nerve fibers.

All these nerve fibers converge, collectively forming the peripheral nerves, before they connect with the brain or spinal cord. Most peripheral nerves from different parts of the body connect to the spinal cord. These are called spinal nerves. Those from the face and head connect directly to the lower parts of the brain or brain stem and are known as cranial nerves (see page 36).

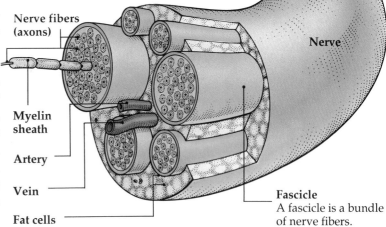

One nerve contains many nerve fibers
A nerve is constructed somewhat like a telephone cable. It consists of numerous nerve fibers, each insulated with a myelin sheath (like individual telephone wires), which are grouped in bundles called fascicles. Each fascicle contains a variety of nerve fibers – sensory, motor, and autonomic – needed to supply a particular location in the body. Fascicles may then split to form different branches of the nerve serving an organ or tissue.

Ganglion
The nerve cell bodies of some of the nerve fibers converge in bulges called ganglia.

Nerve

Nerve fibers (axons)

Myelin sheath

Artery

Vein

Fat cells

Fascicle
A fascicle is a bundle of nerve fibers.

NERVE COMPRESSION

Internal or external pressure can compress nerves against surrounding structures. This constriction reduces blood supply and inhibits function. The effects of a compressed nerve depend on whether the nerve consists of sensory nerve fibers, motor nerve fibers, or both. Possible effects include pain and tingling sensations and numbness. Prolonged compression can cause loss of muscle power and tone, involuntary muscle twitching, and muscle wasting, which are usually restricted to the muscle group supplied by the nerve. Most nerve compression is temporary.

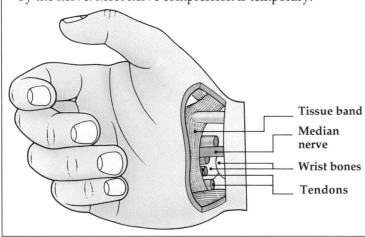

Tissue band

Median nerve

Wrist bones

Tendons

Radial nerve — Humerus

"Saturday night palsy"
External pressure under the armpit can cause compression of the radial nerve. This nerve compression produces temporary paralysis of muscles in the forearm and some sensory impairment in the hand. "Saturday night palsy" is so named because it can occur when a person falls asleep with an arm dangling over the back of a chair, often after excessive drinking.

Wrist pain – is it carpal tunnel syndrome?
This syndrome involves compression of the median nerve as it passes through a tunnel formed by the wrist bones (carpals) and a tight band of tissue that binds the bones together. Tissue swelling inside the tunnel compresses the nerve and causes tingling, intermittent numbness of the thumb and first two fingers, and pain in the forearm. Carpal tunnel syndrome may occur spontaneously or may result from repetitive motion, such as assembly line work.

THE SPINAL NERVES

Between each two adjacent vertebrae, a pair of nerves extends into the body from the spinal cord. Each nerve divides into four branches, or rami; from these branches, nerves divide further to reach all parts of the body.

Cervical spinal nerves (C1 to C8)
These eight pairs of very large nerves supply the neck, back of the head, shoulders, arms and hands, and diaphragm.

Lumbar spinal nerves (L1 to L5)
These five pairs of large nerves supply the lower back and lower abdomen, buttocks, some parts of the external genitalia, and parts of the legs.

Coccygeal spinal nerves
This single pair of very small nerves supplies the skin in the region of the coccyx.

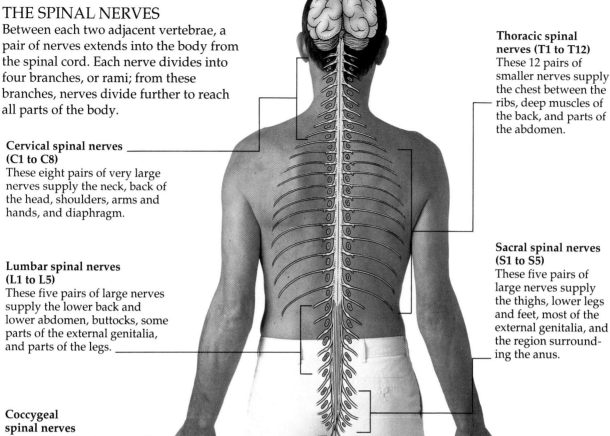

Thoracic spinal nerves (T1 to T12)
These 12 pairs of smaller nerves supply the chest between the ribs, deep muscles of the back, and parts of the abdomen.

Sacral spinal nerves (S1 to S5)
These five pairs of large nerves supply the thighs, lower legs and feet, most of the external genitalia, and the region surrounding the anus.

The dermatomes
Each pair of spinal nerves emerges from a distinct section of the spinal cord and supplies motor, sensory, and autonomic nerve fibers to a localized area of the body, called a dermatome. Each dermatome is coded in the same way as the pair of spinal nerves that supplies it (for example, C2 to C8 and T1 to T12). The arm and leg are each formed from half a dozen extended and developed dermatomes. Loss of sensation or movement in a dermatome indicates the specific spinal nerve that is injured or malfunctioning.

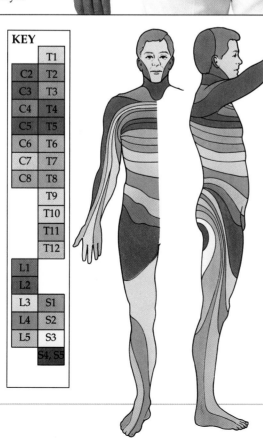

KEY

	T1
C2	T2
C3	T3
C4	T4
C5	T5
C6	T6
C7	T7
C8	T8
	T9
	T10
	T11
	T12
L1	
L2	
L3	S1
L4	S2
L5	S3
	S4, S5

The somatic nervous system

The somatic sensory nerve fibers relay information about skin sensations (see SENSING on page 42), while the somatic motor nerve fibers cause contraction of skeletal muscles (see HOW NERVE SIGNALS CAUSE MUSCLE CONTRACTION on page 32 and MOVING on page 48). Collectively, these nerve fibers form the somatic peripheral nervous system.

The autonomic nervous system

The autonomic nervous system regulates your involuntary bodily functions, such as heart rate and digestion. Motor nerve fibers that regulate internal organs and glands, and sensory nerve fibers that monitor events in the organs, form this division of the peripheral nervous system. The functions of this system are described in Chapter 3 on page 70.

HOW NERVE SIGNALS CAUSE MUSCLE CONTRACTION

Your peripheral nervous system carries signals from your central nervous system to your body's muscles, causing them to contract. Contraction of certain muscles, along with the simultaneous relaxation of opposing muscles, produces all body movement. Volleys of nerve signals carried along motor nerve fibers to the muscles bring about these contractions.

Muscle structure

Each skeletal muscle is made up of bundles of long, thin, cylindrical fibers. They contain bundles of microscopic filaments. When a muscle contracts, these filaments undergo a chemical reaction that causes them to slide over each other. This induces the fibers and the entire muscle to shorten.

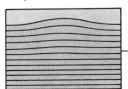

Relaxed muscle

Muscle fibers when relaxed

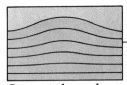

Contracted muscle

Shortened muscle fibers

Lifting an object

When you lift an apple to your mouth, the biceps muscle in the front of your upper arm contracts. At the same time, the opposing triceps muscle in the back of your upper arm relaxes. Nerve signals travel from the brain, down the spinal cord, and along motor nerve fibers in a peripheral nerve to the muscles, causing them to contract.

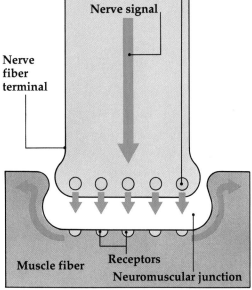

Brain

Spinal cord

Motor nerve fibers

Biceps muscle

Triceps muscle

A muscle's nerve supply

Each muscle fiber receives input from a branch of a single nerve fiber. The force or intensity of muscle contraction depends on the number of nerve fibers and muscle fibers that are activated.

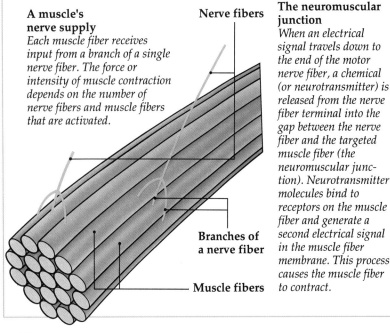

Nerve fibers

Branches of a nerve fiber

Muscle fibers

The neuromuscular junction

When an electrical signal travels down to the end of the motor nerve fiber, a chemical (or neurotransmitter) is released from the nerve fiber terminal into the gap between the nerve fiber and the targeted muscle fiber (the neuromuscular junction). Neurotransmitter molecules bind to receptors on the muscle fiber and generate a second electrical signal in the muscle fiber membrane. This process causes the muscle fiber to contract.

Neurotransmitter

Nerve signal

Nerve fiber terminal

Muscle fiber

Receptors

Neuromuscular junction

SPINAL REFLEXES

A reflex is a predictable, automatic response of the nervous system to an outside event or internal stimulus. Reflexes regulate many internal mechanisms as well as responses to external circumstances. The spinal cord can perform many simple reflexes independently of the brain. Most of these are defense mechanisms to protect against injury, such as withdrawing your hand from a hot surface. Some reflexes, such as blinking your eye, stem from lower portions of the brain that are not involved in conscious thought.

In a fully developed, healthy person, many reflexes can be consciously modified – inhibited or strengthened – by nerve signals that travel down the spinal cord from the cerebral cortex. For example, you can control your urge to urinate. Unmodified reflexes rarely occur if you are conscious and alert. When you are distracted, relaxed, or asleep, however, unmodified reflexes can occur.

If the brain is totally disconnected from the spinal cord and the body is stimulated appropriately, spinal reflexes still occur. This explains the reflex movements during coma and in a person whose spinal cord has been severed.

NEUROPATHIES

A neuropathy is a peripheral nerve disorder that impairs nerve function, leading to numbness, pain, weakness, or paralysis. A neuropathy may involve a single nerve, producing symptoms in a limited area. Multiple nerves can also be damaged in a nerve disorder such as diabetic neuropathy.

Causes
A neuropathy can be caused by several disorders: destruction of nerve cell bodies in the spinal cord, degeneration of the insulating layer of myelin surrounding a nerve, or physical damage or loss of blood

HOW DO REFLEXES WORK?

In a reflex action, a specialized sensory receptor or organ detects a stimulus. The stimulus is then converted into signals that travel along sensory nerve fibers to a central point – the brain or spinal cord. Signals are then generated in motor nerve fibers and carried to a target muscle, organ, or cell. These principles operate in the two spinal reflex actions described below.

THE KNEE-JERK REFLEX

Doctors check this reflex to make sure the pathways up and down your spine are intact.

1 When your doctor taps the patellar tendon in your knee, a muscle in your thigh stretches, causing sensory signals to travel to your spinal cord by way of sensory nerve fibers.

2 Once they have reached your spinal cord, signals are transmitted from sensory nerve fibers to motor nerve fibers and then to your front thigh muscle, causing it to contract. Your knee joint extends, causing a small kick of your leg and foot.

THE BLADDER CONTROL REFLEX

1 As your bladder fills, stretch receptors in the bladder wall trigger sensory signals that travel to your spinal cord via sensory fibers in the pelvic nerves. Signals travel back to the bladder via motor fibers and cause the bladder to contract. Your conscious control may override the reflex, causing contractions to stop until the bladder has filled further.

2 If the reflex is not overridden and the contractions reach a certain level, signals are relayed to the external sphincter muscle, inhibiting muscle contraction and allowing you to release urine from your bladder.

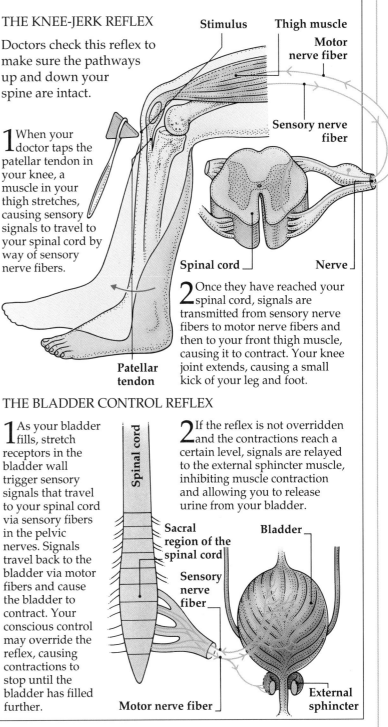

Labels: Stimulus, Thigh muscle, Motor nerve fiber, Sensory nerve fiber, Spinal cord, Nerve, Patellar tendon, Spinal cord, Sacral region of the spinal cord, Sensory nerve fiber, Bladder, Motor nerve fiber, External sphincter

CAUSES OF NEUROPATHY

Some causes of neuropathy include:

◆ Excessive alcohol consumption
◆ Long-standing diabetes mellitus
◆ Deficiencies of such vitamins as thiamine and vitamin B_{12}
◆ Certain cancers
◆ Lead poisoning
◆ Kidney or liver failure
◆ Certain drugs
◆ Autoimmune diseases
◆ Leprosy
◆ Guillain-Barré syndrome
◆ Certain inherited diseases

supply to a nerve. Many possible specific causes exist (see CAUSES OF NEUROPATHY at left). In some cases, doctors never discover the cause. The person's medical history is the key to an accurate diagnosis.

Treatment

Treatment of neuropathies depends on the cause. For example, lead poisoning is treated with drugs that bind to lead and are excreted. Removing the source of lead (often old house paint) so that no more can be ingested prevents further damage. Doctors also attempt to prevent damage to hands and feet that have become insensitive to injury from neuropathy. Damage to a sensory nerve can make a person lose his or her sensation of pain. Some types of neuropathy, such as those caused by advanced lung cancer, are progressive and untreatable.

CUT AND CRUSH NERVE INJURIES

When a nerve is crushed or partially cut, some of its individual nerve cell fibers are also cut or damaged. Alternatively, a nerve may be severed completely, often as a result of an injury, such as a power saw accident or a knife wound.

Crush and partial cut injuries

If only some nerve fibers are cut or damaged, the remaining portion of the nerve acts as a splint. Fibers usually regenerate in channels formed by their original myelin sheaths, the fatty coatings that cover the axons of nerve cells, until they reach their targets, resulting in slow, progressive, but usually complete, recovery of sensation and movement.

LEAD POISONING

Lead can be an occupational hazard in certain industries. Children who eat old, peeling house paint suffer serious effects from lead poisoning, including lowered IQ and mental retardation. Exposure to lead in the air has lessened since leaded gasoline was banned in the US. But drinking water can be contaminated because lead was used in household plumbing until recently. You can reduce your lead exposure from tap water by letting the water run for a few minutes before drinking it.

HOW LEAD AFFECTS THE BODY

Reproductive organs
Lead has serious effects on reproductive organs of men and women, including impotence, sperm damage, miscarriage, stillbirth, and sterility.

Digestive tract

Gastrointestinal effects of lead poisoning include abdominal pain (lead colic), constipation or diarrhea, loss of appetite, nausea, and vomiting.

Kidneys
Kidney disease can develop from lead poisoning. Usually, no symptoms develop until the damage has become irreversible.

Nervous system
Lead affects the entire nervous system. Early signs of lead poisoning are restlessness, sleep disturbances, fatigue, dizziness, headache, memory loss, and tremors. Lead poisoning leads to weakness in the hands and feet.

Lead in the bloodstream
Lead flows to all parts of the body in the bloodstream. It breaks down the blood-brain barrier, allowing some substances that would otherwise be blocked to pass through to the brain.

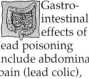

Severed nerve

The individual nerve fibers of a completely severed nerve can regenerate in their original sheaths only if the two ends are precisely reattached. If the ends do not meet, the fibers attempt to regenerate but only form a lump of tissue called a neuroma (a benign tumor).

Under ideal circumstances, surgeons can rejoin the cut ends with microsurgery using delicate sutures and needles. Even with the best surgical repair, however, recovery is rarely complete because regenerating nerve fibers extend into the wrong channels. Restored function may produce unintended actions; for example, an attempt to move the index finger may move the middle finger as well. In some cases, the motor cortex eventually reprograms the areas that control movements and function improves.

NERVE FIBER REGENERATION

A severed nerve fiber can regenerate, provided the nerve cell body, the myelin sheath around the nerve fiber, and the blood supply to the nerve are intact. Such regrowth occurs at the rate of about half an inch every month.

1 After a nerve fiber has been severed, the part farthest from the cell body degenerates.

Cell body **Nerve fiber** **Target**

Myelin sheath **Degenerated part of fiber**

2 The remaining portion of the fiber generates sprouts, one of which begins to extend down the old nerve fiber sheath.

Site of cut

Sprouts

3 The regenerating fiber eventually reaches the original target site of the nerve cell.

Regenerating fiber

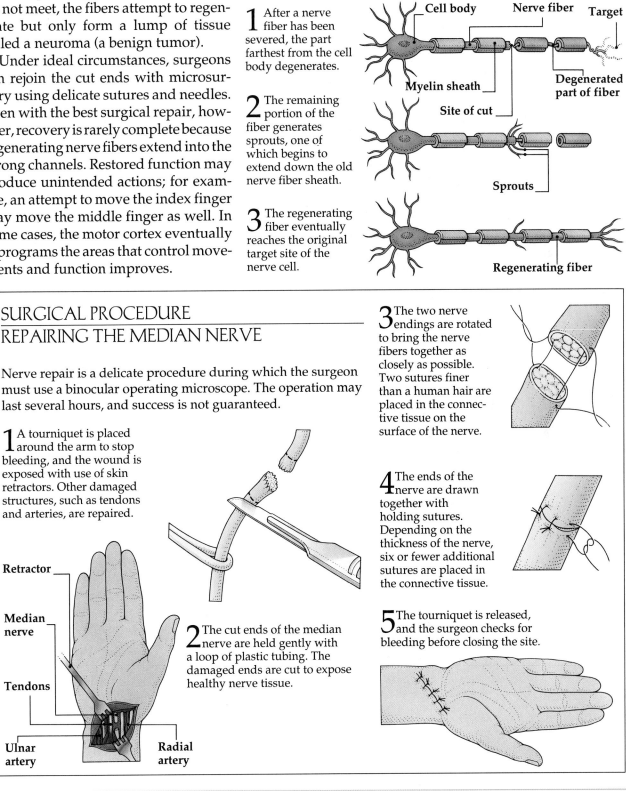

SURGICAL PROCEDURE
REPAIRING THE MEDIAN NERVE

Nerve repair is a delicate procedure during which the surgeon must use a binocular operating microscope. The operation may last several hours, and success is not guaranteed.

1 A tourniquet is placed around the arm to stop bleeding, and the wound is exposed with use of skin retractors. Other damaged structures, such as tendons and arteries, are repaired.

Retractor

Median nerve

Tendons

Ulnar artery

Radial artery

2 The cut ends of the median nerve are held gently with a loop of plastic tubing. The damaged ends are cut to expose healthy nerve tissue.

3 The two nerve endings are rotated to bring the nerve fibers together as closely as possible. Two sutures finer than a human hair are placed in the connective tissue on the surface of the nerve.

4 The ends of the nerve are drawn together with holding sutures. Depending on the thickness of the nerve, six or fewer additional sutures are placed in the connective tissue.

5 The tourniquet is released, and the surgeon checks for bleeding before closing the site.

THE CRANIAL NERVES

The cranial nerves exit the central nervous system from the lower portions of the brain to supply the head, face, neck, shoulders, and some organs. Cranial nerve fibers may mainly contain sensory nerve fibers, or motor nerve fibers, or various combinations of sensory, motor, and autonomic nerve fibers.

The cranial nerves

Among the 12 pairs of cranial nerves, one pair – the olfactory nerves – emerges from the underside of the cerebrum. Another pair – the optic nerves – emerges from the thalamus underneath the brain. The other 10 pairs emerge from the brain stem. Each pair is given a Roman numeral and a name.

Olfactory nerves (I)
Sensory nerve fibers in these nerves are activated by odors that disperse and stimulate receptors high in the nose.

I

Oculomotor nerves (III)
These nerves contain motor nerve fibers that cause eyeball and eye lid movements, change the pupil size, and adjust the lens shape for near vision.

III

Abducens nerves (VI)
These nerves contain motor fibers that control the movement of certain eye muscles.

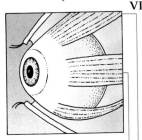

VI

Trochlear nerves (IV)
These nerves contain motor nerve fibers that aid eyeball movement.

IV

Optic nerves (II)
Sensory nerve fibers in these nerves transmit information about visual images received by the retina.

II

Cerebrum

Brain stem

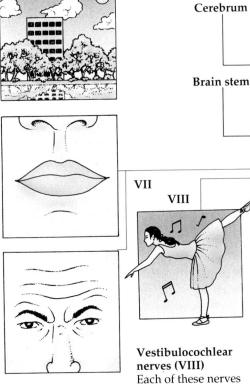

Facial nerves (VII)
Motor fibers in these nerves regulate the muscle movements in facial expressions and the secretion of saliva and tears. Sensory fibers in these nerves relay information about tastes detected by the mouth.

VII

VIII

Spinal cord

XI

XII

Connections with higher brain areas

The cell bodies of the cranial motor nerve fibers are grouped together in localized areas of the brain stem, called motor nuclei. The motor nuclei receive commands from higher areas of the brain to initiate muscle movements. Cranial sensory nerve fibers connect to nerve cell bodies called sensory nuclei in the brain stem. Nerve fibers from the sensory nuclei relay information about sensations in the head, neck, and shoulders to higher areas of the brain. These areas perceive the messages and form a response.

Vestibulocochlear nerves (VIII)
Each of these nerves has two branches. The vestibular branch contains sensory fibers that carry information about body balance and equilibrium from the inner ear. The auditory branch contains sensory fibers that transmit information about sounds.

Spinal accessory nerves (XI)
These nerves contain motor fibers that control movements of certain shoulder and neck muscles.

Hypoglossal nerves (XII)
These nerves contain motor fibers that regulate movements of the tongue that occur during speech and eating.

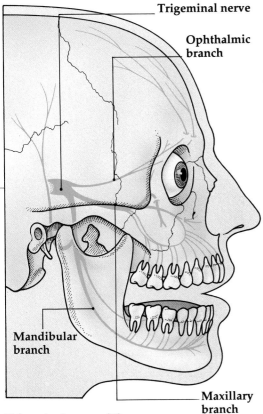

Trigeminal nerve

Ophthalmic branch

Mandibular branch

Maxillary branch

Trigeminal nerves (V)

Each of these nerves has three branches – ophthalmic (eye), maxillary (upper jaw), and mandibular (lower jaw). Sensory fibers in these nerves transmit information about sensations in the head and face. Motor fibers in the mandibular branches control chewing movements.

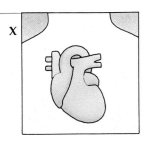

X

Vagus nerves (X)

These nerves contain parasympathetic motor fibers that regulate various functions, such as swallowing, speech production, and heart rate. They also contain sensory fibers that convey information from the larynx, trachea, heart, and other organs.

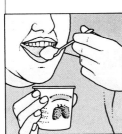

IX

Glossopharyngeal nerves (IX)

Sensory fibers in these nerves provide further information from the mouth about taste. Their motor fibers regulate swallowing movements and the secretion of saliva.

Facial pain

Trigeminal neuralgia is a disorder of the trigeminal nerve that causes excruciating facial pain in the area supplied by the nerve. Although the pain lasts only a few minutes, it is often so severe that it causes involuntary wincing. For this reason, the disorder is often called tic douloureux ("painful twitch").

ACOUSTIC NEUROMA

An acoustic neuroma is a benign (noncancerous) tumor that arises in the glial cells that surround the auditory nerve, causing nerve compression. The initial result is ringing in the ear (tinnitus) and hearing loss. As the tumor enlarges and compresses adjacent nerve tissue, loss of balance, facial pain, or facial weakness may occur. The doctor may confirm the diagnosis using magnetic resonance imaging (MRI). The resulting image, as shown below, reveals the location and size of the tumor (arrow), which is then removed.

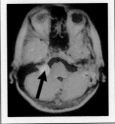

Q **I have had an attack of shingles. Why did it affect only certain areas of my skin?**

A Shingles, which usually produces a painful rash, is caused by the same virus that causes chicken pox. After an attack of chicken pox, the virus lies dormant in the sensory nerve cell bodies of spinal nerves. Under certain conditions, the virus reactivates in some of the sensory nerve cells and produces the shingles rash. Each spinal nerve supplies a certain segment of the body, called a dermatome. The shingles rash only occurs on skin areas within the affected dermatome. Doctors do not know why the virus reactivates in one nerve but not another.

Q **My aunt suffered a severe head injury 6 months ago. She has recovered almost completely but has lost her sense of smell. Is this loss permanent?**

A The sense of smell is controlled by delicate, specialized nerve endings that penetrate the upper bones of the nasal cavities. Severed olfactory nerves do not regenerate easily. Nerves usually regenerate at a rate of about half an inch per month, so if your aunt has not regained her sense of smell by now, she probably will not do so.

Q **My mother had polio as a teenager, which caused some weakness of her leg muscles. Why is her sensation normal?**

A Polio attacks the motor nerve cells of the spinal cord, which control movement. Sensory nerve cells are unaffected by the viral infection, so sensation remains normal.

CHAPTER TWO

THE CONSCIOUS BRAIN

MOST PEOPLE experience life as an ever-changing spectrum of sound and vision, enhanced by touch, taste, and smell. Our thoughts and emotions interpret and react to these perceptions. From these experiences, the human brain synthesizes reality, and we learn how to interact with the outside world. Each of these experiences and abilities is a function of the conscious brain, but the act of defining consciousness itself presents a problem. A good definition includes the awareness we have of ourselves and our surroundings. But this awareness fluctuates from moment to moment. During significant life events, such as the birth of a child, or during moments of danger, we have a keen sense of where we are and what is happening. But when performing a mundane task, such as folding laundry, our mind often wanders and our awareness decreases. During some states, such as sleep, the brain's activity becomes altered but is not necessarily diminished. While dreaming, we sometimes have experiences that seem just as real as those we have while we are awake. In unconscious states, such as coma after a severe head injury, very little brain activity may be present. This chapter discusses the different lev-

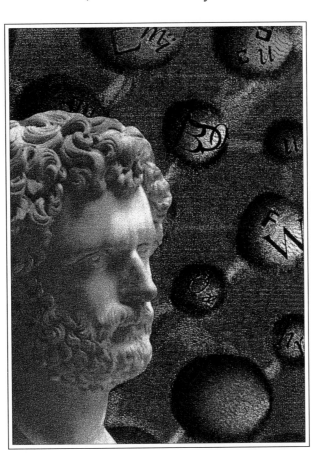

els of consciousness. It also describes your conscious control of movement and use of language as well as your awareness of incoming sensations. The complex system of sensory input that travels to the brain mirrors an equally complex system of outgoing nerve impulses. These impulses control and coordinate your muscles, giving you a high degree of conscious control over your movements and actions.

The chapter goes on to explore the higher functions of the brain that govern the characteristically human abilities of thinking, understanding, and knowing. We can only speculate about the way these functions work. How do we think? What does it mean to understand? Why do we remember some things easily and forget others? Throughout history, philosophers have struggled to understand how the brain receives, analyzes, and interprets information from the senses. Although medical science has made important contributions to this understanding, many questions remain unanswered. But we do know that the brain's ability to understand sensory information, combined with its aptitude for storing information and learning from experience, enable you to make important decisions about actions that shape your life.

CONSCIOUSNESS

CONSCIOUSNESS implies awareness – seeing, hearing, and perceiving the events around you and responding to them. If you are asleep, suffering from a concussion, or under the influence of anesthesia, you are not conscious of the external world and do not respond to it. Life goes on without your participation.

Human consciousness involves more than simple wakefulness. Consciousness includes the self-awareness that provides every human with a sense of personal identity. Conscious awareness also implies memory and the ability to make choices based on past experiences. Being conscious also involves a person's thought, intention, and will, culminating in purposeful action.

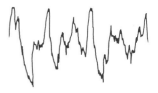

Awake but relaxed

Deep sleep

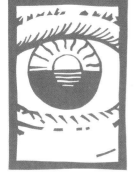

Are animals conscious?
All animals have sensory structures that enable them to be aware of their environment. But animals lack the self-awareness that we possess. Although some primates seem able to recognize their own reflections, higher intellectual functions, such as abstract thought, are absent.

Signals from active reticular formation radiate to cortex

Cerebral cortex

Visual impulses activate reticular formation

How do we maintain consciousness?
We maintain awareness through the reticular activating system – the arousal system – illustrated here. The reticular activating system is a complex pathway of nerve cells that originates in an area of the brain stem called the reticular formation and continues through the thalamus and hypothalamus to the cerebral cortex. The activity level in the reticular system determines a person's level of awareness of thought processes, the external world, and bodily functions.

Auditory impulses activate reticular formation

Impulses from spinal cord activate reticular formation

Reticular formation

Levels of consciousness
There are many levels of consciousness, from deep sleep to the acute alertness needed to play a video game. Each level displays a characteristic type of electrical activity in the brain and this brain activity can be measured. Electrodes placed on the scalp record the brain's electrical output in the form of a wave pattern called an electroencephalogram (EEG). The EEG reflects the state of neural activity in the brain. The upper waveform shown above is an alpha wave, which occurs when a person is awake but relaxed with eyes closed. Alpha waves also occur during states of hypnosis and meditation. The lower waveform is a delta wave, seen in deep sleep.

CONTROL OF UNCONSCIOUS FUNCTIONS

Much of our primitive, "animal" brain activity lies beyond conscious control. Our body temperature and heart rate are regulated automatically by the autonomic nervous system. However, studies have shown that humans can achieve some control of unconscious bodily functions.

The influence of meditation
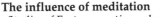
Studies of Eastern mystics and yoga practitioners have confirmed that a remarkable degree of control over bodily functions is possible. Some yogis have been able to survive such physical trials as being buried alive or being exposed to extreme heat or cold.

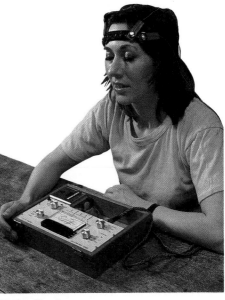

Biofeedback
Biofeedback has been used to control heart rate or blood pressure. Instruments record the body's output and feed the information to the subject, who learns to alter the readings at will. Sometimes subjects are then able to alter their heart rate or blood pressure without the equipment.

WHAT MAKES HUMANS CONSCIOUS?

The brains of all mammals and most reptiles are similar in structure. All have regions that control basic bodily functions and movements, such as fixing the eyes on a moving object and tracking it. But when body weight is considered, the size of the cerebral cortex varies substantially among species. This variation reflects the different information-processing capacities of each species (see EVOLUTION AND DEVELOPMENT on page 12). Intelligence and complexity of thought increase with the size of the "thinking" structures of the brain. Fully conscious awareness also involves the ability to "construct reality." Understanding the outside world and your place within it is a uniquely human ability. Only a few animals other than humans – chimpanzees and orangutans – can even understand their reflection in a mirror. Animal behavior is driven by reflexes and instincts, but humans have choice. In circumstances that require decision making, your brain relies on its vast storehouse of memories to call up a like event, remember your response, and recall whether the outcome was desirable. Your brain helps you decide whether to respond as you did before or in a new way.

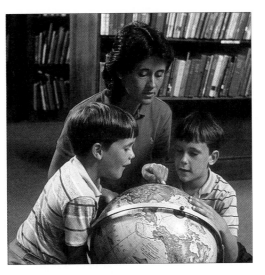

Learning and memory
The ability to evaluate information and learn from experience is more highly developed in humans than in any other animal species. When coupled with our ability to transmit experience from one generation to the next, this ability contributes to the continued growth of human knowledge.

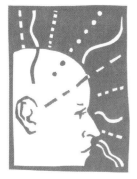

SENSING

Y OUR ABILITY to detect, interpret, and respond to the continual bombardment of information from the environment depends on the normal functioning of your senses. Without taste, touch, smell, hearing, and sight, you would be entirely cut off from incoming external impressions. But your body also responds to internally generated sensations, such as body temperature.

SENSORY DEPRIVATION

Experiments have shown that we need continuous sensory stimulation to maintain normal functioning. During these experiments, people who were deprived of all sensory stimulation frequently hallucinated and were sometimes unable to distinguish between sleeping and waking. Such findings suggest that when we are deprived of sensory information, the brain compensates by generating fantasies that may turn into overpowering sensory illusions.

Any change in the external or internal environment can be a stimulus to your nervous system. Your body's sensory receptors detect a stimulus and convert it into signals that travel to the central nervous system by means of sensory nerve cells. Your brain analyzes these signals and decides whether or not to bring them to your conscious attention.

SENSORY RECEPTORS

Some sensory receptors are for taste, smell, hearing, vision, and balance. Others are linked to touch, temperature, pressure, and pain, which originate on the body's surface. These sensations also include pain or pressure from the internal organs, such as angina (heart pain) and sensations that provide information about the body's position. Receptors for sight,

The human sensory system
Compared with the sensory capacities of some lower animals, the sensory ability of humans may be unremarkable. Your dog's sense of smell is 1 million times greater than yours for some odors because the dog's olfactory membrane and portions of the brain devoted to the sense of smell (olfaction) are more highly developed.

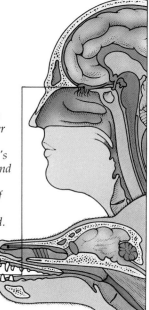

Olfactory membrane

hearing, smell, and taste lie in the retinas of the eyes, in the inner ears, in the upper back of the nose, and on the tongue's surface. These receptors transmit signals directly to the brain.

The "five senses"
The Greek philosopher Aristotle established the concept of the five senses – sight, hearing, touch, smell, and taste. Without these senses, we cannot fully relate to the environment. The human sensory system also perceives many internal stimuli, such as a sense of imbalance.

SENSORY PATHWAYS TO THE BRAIN

The diagram below depicts the pathway of sensory signals sent from the different sensory organs and receptors throughout the body, their final destination in the brain, and the senses for which they are responsible. The colored blocks correspond to the areas of the brain indicated at right.

Taste area
Visual area
Cerebellum
Brain stem
Spinal cord

General sensory area
Thalamus
Limbic system
Hearing area

Sensory areas of cerebral cortex

Spinal cord

Muscle and joint receptors

Eyes

Cerebellum

Thalamus

Internal organs

Brain stem

Balance organs in ears
Cochleas in ears

Vision
Position
Hearing
Touch, pain, and temperature
Taste

Skin

Tongue

Nose

Limbic system

Receptors for touch sensations are located just under the skin's surface, in muscles and joints, and in the internal organs. They relay their signals to the brain stem or to the spinal cord. From these regions, the signals may be sent to higher areas of the brain.

SENSORY PATHWAYS

Sensory nerve cells receive and convey signals from different sensory organs and receptors. In the spinal cord, these nerve cells create pathways that lead to their ultimate targets (see SENSORY PATHWAYS TO THE BRAIN above).

Impulses from somatic receptors enter the spinal cord through the dorsal (back) roots of spinal nerves. There they may be relayed to other nerve cells that send their fibers up the spinal cord. These fibers form cablelike structures called tracts. The ascending tracts carry signals from the sensory receptors upward toward the brain. Descending tracts

Touch sensation

The illustration below shows what you might look like if your body were proportioned according to the amount of cerebral cortex devoted to each body part's sensory input. The large amount of cerebral cortex devoted to certain body parts, such as the face, hands, or genitals (not pictured), is a product of evolution and has helped the human species survive during its long history.

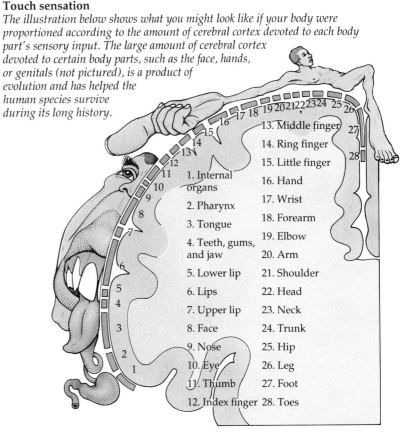

13. Middle finger
14. Ring finger
15. Little finger
16. Hand
17. Wrist
18. Forearm
19. Elbow
20. Arm
21. Shoulder
22. Head
23. Neck
24. Trunk
25. Hip
26. Leg
27. Foot
28. Toes

1. Internal organs
2. Pharynx
3. Tongue
4. Teeth, gums, and jaw
5. Lower lip
6. Lips
7. Upper lip
8. Face
9. Nose
10. Eye
11. Thumb
12. Index finger

SENSORY RECEPTORS IN THE SKIN

The skin is your body's largest sensory organ. It contains a vast array of sensory receptors. These receptors may be located close to the skin's surface or in deeper layers.

Some receptors are enclosed in capsules. Others are not. Encapsulated receptors respond to low-level stimulation; uncovered receptors respond to pain and temperature.

Meissner's corpuscle
This encapsulated receptor, shown below (magnified 200 times), lies close to the skin's surface, particularly in the lips and hands. These corpuscles respond to gentle touch and low-frequency vibration.

Free nerve ending
Touch, pressure, and pain receptor

Merkel's disk
Touch and pressure receptor

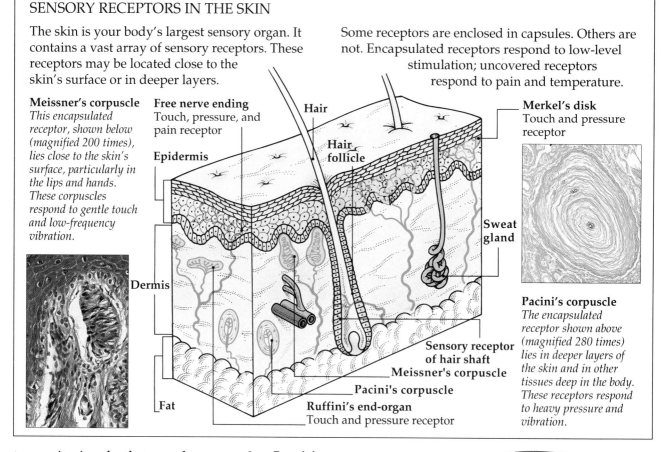

Hair

Hair follicle

Epidermis

Dermis

Fat

Sweat gland

Sensory receptor of hair shaft

Meissner's corpuscle

Pacini's corpuscle

Ruffini's end-organ
Touch and pressure receptor

Pacini's corpuscle
The encapsulated receptor shown above (magnified 280 times) lies in deeper layers of the skin and in other tissues deep in the body. These receptors respond to heavy pressure and vibration.

transmit signals that produce muscle contraction or glandular secretion. Different ascending tracts in the spinal cord carry specific types of sensory information. Some carry impulses for pressure, pain, temperature, and sense of position. These tracts form part of a large, highly specialized sensory pathway. Single nerve cells in these tracts respond to only one type of stimulus. Fibers in these tracts carry touch impulses that tell the brain exactly where the body is touched. Impulses from receptors in moving joints convey messages about different body positions.

When they reach the brain, most impulses conveying somatic sensation pass first to the thalamus and then to two regions of the cortex called the somatosensory cortices. Other signals pass to the cerebellum (especially signals conveying sense of position) or to the limbic system (signals conveying the emotional aspects of physical pain).

Perceiving sensations: your body's telephone system
Multiple receptors under your skin receive impulses the same way a telephone receiver does. These receptors act as the receiving end of a nerve line that then sends a message into your spinal cord. Impulses from different types of stimuli – an ice cube or the touch of a feather – travel up the spinal cord along different cables, or tracts. These impulses sometimes cross in the spinal cord but all end in the thalamus, which relays the sensory impulses to your sensory cortex. Your brain responds to the stimulus and prompts an outgoing "telephone message" that tells your body how to react.

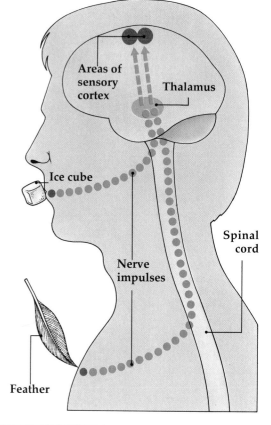

Areas of sensory cortex

Thalamus

Ice cube

Nerve impulses

Spinal cord

Feather

THE SPECIAL SENSES

Smell, taste, sight, and hearing, together with the sense of balance detected by the inner ear, are known as the special senses. Although these senses operate largely independently, they can interact with or compensate for each other to provide the brain with needed information. For example, when a person loses the sense of sight, hearing often improves; a person with a hearing disorder learns to rely more heavily on sight. The sense of taste is strongly influenced by odors. The aroma of food travels into the nasal cavities, where it triggers sensitive receptors that enhance taste. This explains why you can't taste food when your nose is congested from a cold.

Our special senses depend on highly specialized sensory organs, but they also rely on the workings of specific areas in the brain. The sensory tissues of the special sense organs – the retina in the eye, the cochlea and semicircular canals in the inner ear, the olfactory apparatus in the nose, and the taste buds on the tongue – are more susceptible to damage and disease than the brain. But disorders that affect the brain can cause total loss of a special sense.

How do we see?
Rays of light enter the eye and converge on the retina, a light-sensitive layer at the back of each eye. Retinal receptor cells respond to visual information and transmit signals to the brain via the optic nerve. Signals fall on the right and left sides of each retina and are channeled to the corresponding side of the brain. This process requires half the nerve fibers to cross paths at an intersection called the optic chiasm, located at the base of the brain. Damage to an optic tract behind this point affects vision in both eyes.

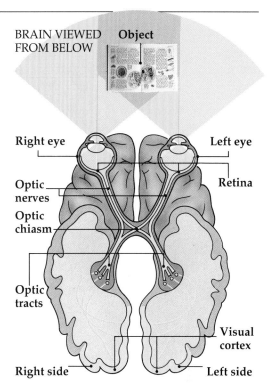

BRAIN VIEWED FROM BELOW   Object

Right eye   Left eye

Optic nerves   Retina

Optic chiasm

Optic tracts

Visual cortex

Right side   Left side

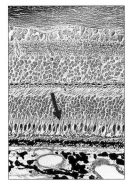

Cross-section through the retina
As seen at left, the retina contains different layers that hold various types of nerve cells. The sensory receptors (known as rods and cones), which translate light into nerve impulses, are located in one of these layers (arrow).

How do we hear?
Sound waves enter the ear, causing the eardrum to vibrate. These vibrations move toward the cochlea, where the vibrations set the basilar membrane in motion, resulting in temporary distortion of hair cells lining the sound receptor. The hair cells stimulate sensory nerve fibers and translate degrees of vibration into impulses that travel to the auditory cortex. This area of the brain can distinguish auditory signals, interpreting them as sounds as diverse as a symphony or a barking dog.

Outer ear

Middle ear

Inner ear

Auditory cortex

Eardrum

Sound waves

Cochlea

Nerve fibers of the cochlear nerve

Hairs   Hair cell

Basilar membrane

Sound wave

TASTE AND SMELL WORK TOGETHER

The way we taste and smell things is only beginning to be understood. Both senses rely on the receptors in the nasal and oral cavities, which respond to chemicals in food or airborne particles. Our sense of smell helps warn us of dangers, such as smoke or spoiled food. Our ability to smell can also evoke emotionally charged memories. Loss of the sense of smell impairs our enjoyment of food. Our tongue can only distinguish sweet, sour, bitter, and salty tastes. Much of what we perceive as taste is actually smell. The sense of smell deteriorates in many people as they age.

PAIN

Pain is your body's way of telling you something is wrong. It is a protective mechanism that alerts your brain to tissue injury and damage. Your perception of pain is influenced by physical sensation and emotion. First, you sense the pain's location in your body. You also feel the type of pain – whether it is sharp, dull, pinching, or burning. Second, you experience the emotional response that accompanies the physical sensation.

Pain receptors

Pain receptors respond to a variety of stimuli. Some respond only to pressure, some to high temperatures, and some to the stimulation of chemicals released by damaged tissue. Other receptors respond to more than one type of stimulation. They respond more broadly, indicating the presence of a dangerous stimulus but not clarifying its type or intensity.

Once stimulated, a receptor transmits pain signals via sensory nerve fibers and the spinal cord to the brain, where you perceive the pain.

PAIN RELIEF

You can usually relieve mild pain caused by a headache or toothache by taking a mild, non-narcotic, analgesic drug, such as aspirin or acetaminophen. Treatment of severe pain from a serious injury or relief of pain after surgery may require narcotic drugs, such as morphine.

Doctors often use local anesthetics to prevent pain during dental procedures or minor operations. To treat chronic pain, doctors sometimes place electrodes on the skin to try to suppress transmission of pain signals to the brain. This technique is not always effective in relieving the pain.

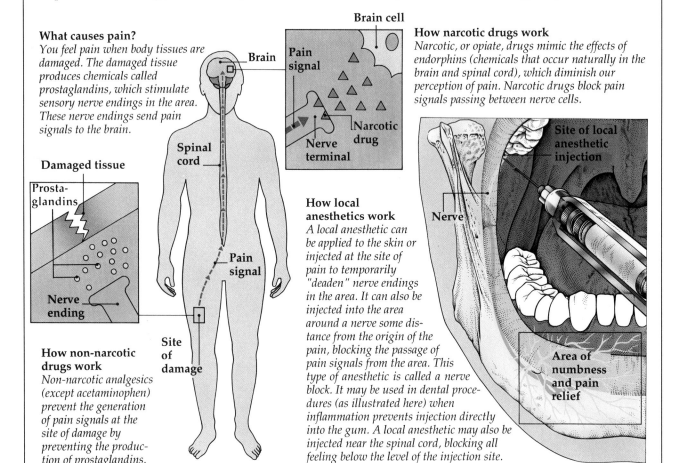

What causes pain?
You feel pain when body tissues are damaged. The damaged tissue produces chemicals called prostaglandins, which stimulate sensory nerve endings in the area. These nerve endings send pain signals to the brain.

Brain

Damaged tissue

Prosta-glandins

Nerve ending

How non-narcotic drugs work
Non-narcotic analgesics (except acetaminophen) prevent the generation of pain signals at the site of damage by preventing the production of prostaglandins.

Spinal cord

Pain signal

Site of damage

Brain cell

Pain signal

Narcotic drug

Nerve terminal

How local anesthetics work
A local anesthetic can be applied to the skin or injected at the site of pain to temporarily "deaden" nerve endings in the area. It can also be injected into the area around a nerve some distance from the origin of the pain, blocking the passage of pain signals from the area. This type of anesthetic is called a nerve block. It may be used in dental procedures (as illustrated here) when inflammation prevents injection directly into the gum. A local anesthetic may also be injected near the spinal cord, blocking all feeling below the level of the injection site.

How narcotic drugs work
Narcotic, or opiate, drugs mimic the effects of endorphins (chemicals that occur naturally in the brain and spinal cord), which diminish our perception of pain. Narcotic drugs block pain signals passing between nerve cells.

Site of local anesthetic injection

Nerve

Area of numbness and pain relief

REFERRED PAIN

Our internal organs have relatively few pain receptors. This explains why internal discomfort and pain is sometimes difficult to identify and locate. Internal pain is sometimes perceived as originating from a body surface some distance from the affected organ, as in an attack of angina (see below). This is called referred pain. It occurs because nerve fibers from the body surface and from the affected internal organ often converge on the same sensory pathways. Sometimes pain may be referred from parts of the body other than organs. For example, a toothache may cause pain in the ear and arthritis in the knee is sometimes felt as pain in the hip.

Angina
During an attack of angina, pain sometimes radiates down the left arm, although the pain originates in the heart.

Reacting to pain

Pain messages are modified within the nervous system. For example, the nervous system contains a highly efficient pain suppression mechanism, which explains why you may not notice an injury you receive during a game of handball until after the game.

The nervous system modulates the experience of pain signals by releasing endorphins, chemicals that block the transmission of pain signals. Opiate drugs, such as morphine, mimic the pain-suppressing effects of endorphins and act at exactly the same sites in the nervous system.

Pain suppression
After an injury, you can sometimes relieve pain by rubbing the injured part. Rubbing stimulates numerous sensory receptors, and the resulting barrage of signals makes it difficult for your brain to detect pain.

ASK YOUR DOCTOR
PAIN

Q Where does pain occur – in the affected part of the body or only in the brain?

A Pain is perceived and exists only in the brain, although its source is in the affected body part. This concept is illustrated by the phenomenon of "phantom" limb pain in which pain is perceived to originate from part of a limb that has been amputated, such as the foot. The pain clearly exists in the brain, although its source is nerve endings in the remaining limb stump.

Q When my sister has a headache, she seems able to cope with the pain much better than I can when I have one. Why is this?

A Studies show that people vary greatly in their ability to tolerate pain. People subjected to the same type of pain also vary in their reaction to it. Two people can interpret the same level of pain very differently. The cause of this difference can be a physical variance in the threshold of pain perception from person to person. Psychological factors can also alter the response to a painful stimulus.

Q Why do I feel so good after jogging? Is it just the satisfaction of knowing that I'm staying in shape or is there a physical cause?

A When you engage in vigorous exercise, such as jogging, your brain produces endorphins, which make you feel euphoric. This phenomenon is called "runner's high." Euphoria, the emotional opposite of suffering, arises from the blockage by endorphins of pain signals in parts of the brain that control emotion.

MOVING

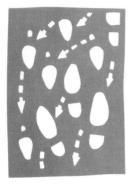

MOST OF US are able to perform everyday activities, such as walking, eating, speaking, and lifting objects, quickly and easily with little awareness of the intricate processes occurring in our bodies. But much of our ability to navigate through our environment, react to stimuli, and manipulate objects involves conscious control over voluntary movements.

Newly acquired and complicated skills, such as driving, require concentration and practice before we can perform them easily. The advanced skills of a trapeze artist require the coordination of movement with a keen sense of timing. These movements demand the synchronized activity of specialized areas of the brain.

5 Peripheral nerves

The spinal motor nerve cell fibers exit the spinal cord and travel in the peripheral nerves.

PLANNING A MOVEMENT

Before you can perform a consciously controlled movement, such as picking up a fork, your brain must form a coordinated plan of action so that all your muscles and other parts of your body move together. This plan, called the central motor program, emerges from association areas of the cerebral cortex. These areas instantaneously "decide" which sets of muscles you will use – in this case, the muscles needed to extend your arm and bring your fingers together to pick up the

6 Skeletal muscles

The instructions reach their final destination: the skeletal muscle fibers. These fibers respond by contracting or relaxing to bring about a voluntary movement. Each spinal motor nerve cell acts on certain muscle fibers.

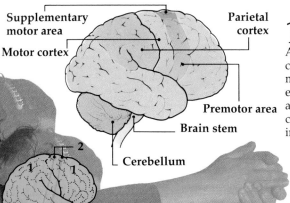

Supplementary
motor area

Motor cortex

Parietal
cortex

Premotor area

Brain stem

Cerebellum

**1 The move-
ment plan**
A plan of movement, called the central motor program, evolves in association areas of the cerebral cortex. These areas include the supplementary motor areas, the premotor areas, and areas of the parietal cortex.

2 Motor cortex
Information about the movement plan travels by direct nerve fiber connections to nerve cells of the brain's motor cortex. Motor nerve cells then instruct the skeletal muscles to contract.

Instructions from the premotor and parietal cortices
Information also travels from motor nerve cells in the premotor cortex and areas of the parietal cortex to instruct the skeletal muscles.

Brain areas beneath the cortex
Structures under the cortex, such as the basal ganglia, the cerebellum, and the brain stem, control different aspects of voluntary movement, such as its planning, initiation, updating, and coordination.

4 Motor nerve cells of the spinal cord
The brain transmits instructions to lower motor nerve cells through the spinal cord. The descending motor pathways activate these spinal motor nerve cells.

3 Descending motor tracts
Nerve cells that originate in the cortex, and in some areas beneath the cortex, transmit signals via long nerve fibers that are located in the spinal cord. These nerve fibers form tracts that control the spinal cord's lower motor nerve cells.

PROBLEMS OF HAND-EYE COORDINATION

Your brain uses visual information to monitor and control movements. Visual association areas process the information, which is incorporated into the motor plan. Damage to part of the parietal cortex or premotor areas renders the motor cortex incapable of using this information. People who have this problem, called optic ataxia, find it difficult to coordinate movements with visual information. Such people have normal vision and control over arm movements, but they cannot reach out and touch an object they see.

Learning to control movements
Young children must learn to coordinate hand (and other) movements with visual information before they can perform voluntary movements quickly and accurately. Adults take this ability for granted.

fork. Information about the proposed action travels to nerve cells of the motor cortex, which then instruct individual skeletal muscle fibers about the planned movement toward the fork. The muscles respond by contracting around the fork so that you can grasp it.

THE BRAIN'S MAP OF THE BODY

Motor nerve cells that originate in one side, or hemisphere, of the brain stimulate muscles on the opposite side of the body. This relationship between the motor cortex and muscle groups explains why a stroke in one side of the brain affects muscles on the other side of the body. Certain areas of the motor cortex control certain muscle groups, creating a "map" of the body within the brain (see illustration at right). Muscle groups that are involved in fine motor skills (such as those in the face and hands) are represented by disproportionately large areas of the motor cortex. This map of the body extends to the premotor cortex and supplementary motor areas of the brain, which contain nerve cells that relay information to corresponding body areas in the motor cortex. This is how nerve cells of the motor cortex become activated before muscle contraction.

HOW DOES THE CORTEX CONTROL MOVEMENT?

The cerebral cortex monitors every movement as you make it. For example, if you are riding a bicycle, sensory areas of the cortex continuously receive feedback from your leg muscles. This information then travels back to the premotor cortex, which updates the motor plan to keep all movements on course.

The motor cortex also forms "motor memories" for rapid, skilled movements, such as typing and piano playing. You must perform such movements slowly at first, because your brain needs sen-

A motor map
Each part of the body is represented by a specific area of the motor cortex. Some muscle groups claim a disproportionately large area of the brain. This illustration shows the size various body parts would be if they were as large or as small as the area of the motor cortex that controls them.

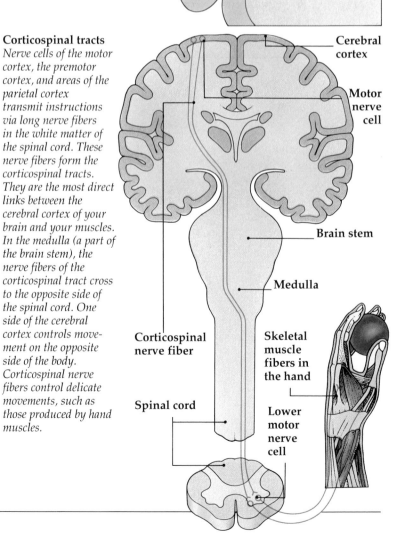

1. Chewing
2. Swallowing
3. Tongue
4. Jaw
5. Vocalization
6. Lips
7. Face
8. Eye
9. Brow
10. Neck
11. Thumb
12. Index finger
13. Middle finger
14. Ring finger
15. Little finger
16. Hand
17. Wrist
18. Elbow
19. Shoulder
20. Trunk
21. Hip
22. Knee
23. Ankle
24. Toes

Corticospinal tracts
Nerve cells of the motor cortex, the premotor cortex, and areas of the parietal cortex transmit instructions via long nerve fibers in the white matter of the spinal cord. These nerve fibers form the corticospinal tracts. They are the most direct links between the cerebral cortex of your brain and your muscles. In the medulla (a part of the brain stem), the nerve fibers of the corticospinal tract cross to the opposite side of the spinal cord. One side of the cerebral cortex controls movement on the opposite side of the body. Corticospinal nerve fibers control delicate movements, such as those produced by hand muscles.

Cerebral cortex

Motor nerve cell

Brain stem

Medulla

Corticospinal nerve fiber

Spinal cord

Skeletal muscle fibers in the hand

Lower motor nerve cell

WRITER'S CRAMP

This painful muscle spasm most often occurs during middle age. A condition similar to writer's cramp sometimes follows the performance of highly skilled motor acts other than writing, such as piano or violin playing. In all cases, a delicate motor skill perfected through years of practice suddenly requires labored, conscious effort. Writer's cramp does not refer to the normal pain most of us feel after holding a pen or pencil for too long. The cause of writer's cramp has been studied extensively with inconclusive results, but experts generally agree that the painful condition is genuine. Doctors usually treat the problem with medication that relieves the cramping.

A painful muscle spasm
When a person who has writer's cramp attempts to write, the thumb, palm, and finger muscles contract into a spasm or become stiff and painful. The spasm sometimes lasts a long time and may spread to the arm and even the shoulder. The spasm disappears only when the person stops trying to write.

HOW DO MUSCLE PAIRS WORK TOGETHER?

Muscles come in pairs – as one muscle contracts, its opposite must relax to bring about movement. Coordinating this contraction and relaxation is very important in voluntary movement and is achieved by the activation of motor nerve cells that tell the muscles how to respond.

sory feedback to guide your muscles through each step. Repeated performance of the same movement (such as practicing musical passages on the piano or letter combinations on a typewriter) creates a lasting memory in your motor cortex. The cortex "remembers" which sequence of nerve cells must be activated to generate the precise sequence of muscle contractions needed to perform the action. Once the motor memory has been formed, you can perform the skilled movement rapidly, with less dependence on sensory feedback.

The supplementary motor area is one of the association areas of the cortex in which your brain develops a movement plan. This area organizes the patterns of nervous system activity you require to perform complex movements, such as opening or closing your hand. Such complicated movements require the coordination of many different groups of muscles in the proper sequence.

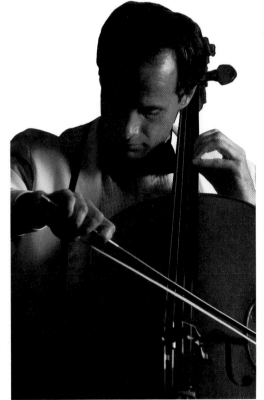

Practice makes perfect
When you start to learn rapid, skilled movements, such as those needed to play a musical instrument, your cortex forms "motor memories" through repeated performance of the movements involved. You must pay close attention to each movement while learning the skill, but once these motor memories are ingrained, you can perform these actions almost automatically. When fully mastered, these movements proceed with speed and grace.

CONTROL OF MOVEMENT, POSTURE, AND BALANCE

The cerebellum, which is located beneath the cerebrum at the back of the brain stem, coordinates movements and controls posture and balance. To accomplish this, it must coordinate its activities with many other areas of the brain. The cerebellum coordinates information about the movement plan, which comes from the motor areas of the cortex, with sensory information about the progress of the movement, which comes from the muscles. By comparing these messages, the cerebellum adjusts the movement as it evolves, keeping it on target. The cerebellum corrects movements in two ways. First, it adjusts the activity of motor nerve cells in the spinal cord, which directly affect the muscles. Second, it continually updates the central motor program.

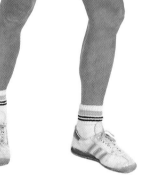

Rapid, accurate movements
The cerebellum is particularly important for the precise execution of rapid, accurate movements – such as those involved in a fast-paced game of ping-pong – that have not been previously practiced.

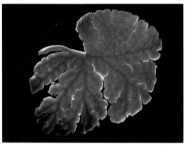

The cerebellum
The photograph at left is a stained section of a slice of cerebellum that shows its delicate structure.

PROBLEMS OF COORDINATION AND BALANCE

Movements can occur if the cerebellum is not functioning, but they display characteristic abnormalities. Damage to the cerebellum destroys the normal, smooth coordination (contraction and relaxation) of opposing muscles. Movements become uncoordinated and jerky. Problems initiating and terminating movements occur: an arm or a leg may overshoot or stop short of its goal. This difficulty, called ataxia, results in an unsteady gait. People with ataxia also have less muscle tone while at rest and display limb tremor during movement, which is most obvious at the end of a movement. Unlike injury to the cerebral cortex, damage to the cerebellum affects muscles on the same side of the body.

An unsteady gait
Damage to the cerebellum causes a characteristic gait marked by a wide stance, unsteady walking, and a tendency to topple.

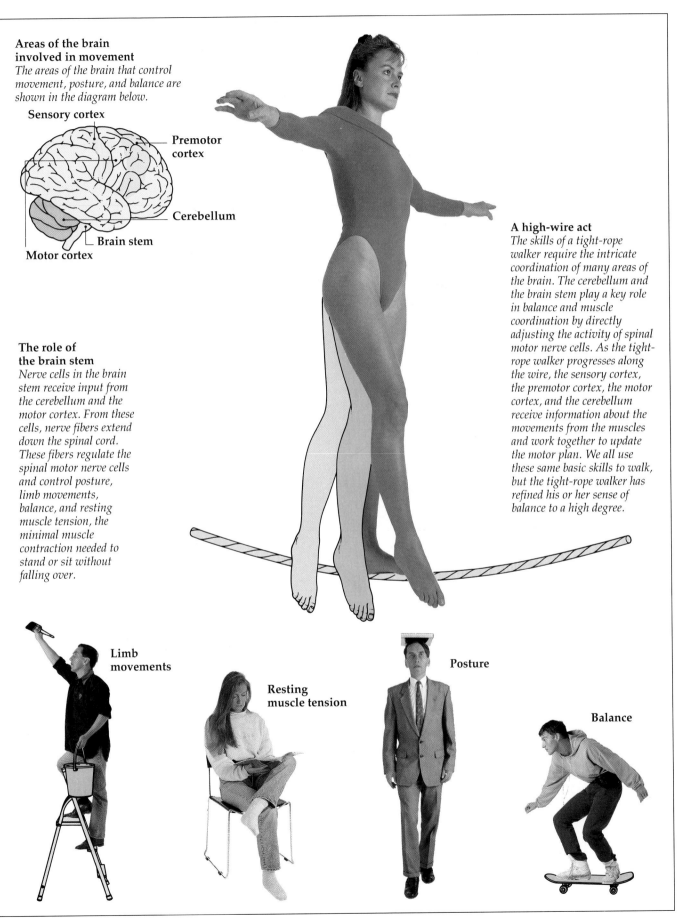

Areas of the brain involved in movement
The areas of the brain that control movement, posture, and balance are shown in the diagram below.

Sensory cortex

Premotor cortex

Cerebellum

Brain stem

Motor cortex

The role of the brain stem
Nerve cells in the brain stem receive input from the cerebellum and the motor cortex. From these cells, nerve fibers extend down the spinal cord. These fibers regulate the spinal motor nerve cells and control posture, limb movements, balance, and resting muscle tension, the minimal muscle contraction needed to stand or sit without falling over.

A high-wire act
The skills of a tight-rope walker require the intricate coordination of many areas of the brain. The cerebellum and the brain stem play a key role in balance and muscle coordination by directly adjusting the activity of spinal motor nerve cells. As the tight-rope walker progresses along the wire, the sensory cortex, the premotor cortex, the motor cortex, and the cerebellum receive information about the movements from the muscles and work together to update the motor plan. We all use these same basic skills to walk, but the tight-rope walker has refined his or her sense of balance to a high degree.

Limb movements

Resting muscle tension

Posture

Balance

MONITOR YOUR SYMPTOMS
TWITCHING AND TREMBLING

Sometimes a part of the body begins twitching involuntarily. This can be frightening if you do not know the cause. Twitching or shaking generally is not serious and usually arises from fatigue or stress. But sometimes these symptoms hint of an underlying condition that requires medical attention.

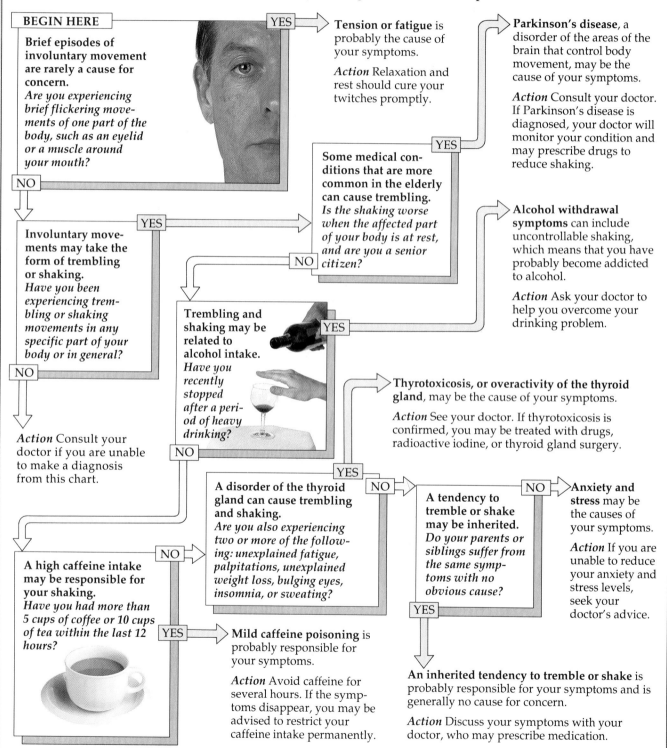

BEGIN HERE

Brief episodes of involuntary movement are rarely a cause for concern.
Are you experiencing brief flickering movements of one part of the body, such as an eyelid or a muscle around your mouth?

NO

YES

Tension or fatigue is probably the cause of your symptoms.

Action Relaxation and rest should cure your twitches promptly.

YES

Involuntary movements may take the form of trembling or shaking.
Have you been experiencing trembling or shaking movements in any specific part of your body or in general?

NO

YES

Some medical conditions that are more common in the elderly can cause trembling.
Is the shaking worse when the affected part of your body is at rest, and are you a senior citizen?

NO

YES

Parkinson's disease, a disorder of the areas of the brain that control body movement, may be the cause of your symptoms.

Action Consult your doctor. If Parkinson's disease is diagnosed, your doctor will monitor your condition and may prescribe drugs to reduce shaking.

Alcohol withdrawal symptoms can include uncontrollable shaking, which means that you have probably become addicted to alcohol.

Action Ask your doctor to help you overcome your drinking problem.

Trembling and shaking may be related to alcohol intake.
Have you recently stopped after a period of heavy drinking?

YES

NO

Thyrotoxicosis, or overactivity of the thyroid gland, may be the cause of your symptoms.

Action See your doctor. If thyrotoxicosis is confirmed, you may be treated with drugs, radioactive iodine, or thyroid gland surgery.

Action Consult your doctor if you are unable to make a diagnosis from this chart.

YES

A disorder of the thyroid gland can cause trembling and shaking.
Are you also experiencing two or more of the following: unexplained fatigue, palpitations, unexplained weight loss, bulging eyes, insomnia, or sweating?

NO

NO

A tendency to tremble or shake may be inherited.
Do your parents or siblings suffer from the same symptoms with no obvious cause?

YES

NO

Anxiety and stress may be the causes of your symptoms.

Action If you are unable to reduce your anxiety and stress levels, seek your doctor's advice.

A high caffeine intake may be responsible for your shaking.
Have you had more than 5 cups of coffee or 10 cups of tea within the last 12 hours?

NO

YES

Mild caffeine poisoning is probably responsible for your symptoms.

Action Avoid caffeine for several hours. If the symptoms disappear, you may be advised to restrict your caffeine intake permanently.

An inherited tendency to tremble or shake is probably responsible for your symptoms and is generally no cause for concern.

Action Discuss your symptoms with your doctor, who may prescribe medication.

THE BASAL GANGLIA

The basal ganglia are paired nerve cell clusters deep within the cerebrum and upper brain stem. They plan, initiate, and control complex patterns and sequences of learned movements, particularly slow, steady movements, such as walking. Their structures are interconnected by many nerve fiber pathways. Nerve cells from all areas of the cerebral cortex send nerve fibers to the basal ganglia. The basal ganglia transmit messages back to the cortex by way of the thalamus to regulate motor functions of the cortex. The normal functioning of all these connections is vital for the smooth control of voluntary movements.

Basal ganglia disorders

When the basal ganglia malfunction, control of voluntary movement suffers. For example, in Parkinson's disease, some neural connections containing the neurotransmitter dopamine fail. Signs of the disease include a tremor of the hands when resting and muscle rigidity. Movements become difficult to initiate and can only be performed slowly (see page 116 for details).

In Huntington's chorea, a hereditary disorder, nerve cells containing the neurotransmitter gamma-aminobutyric acid (GABA) degenerate. This causes uncontrollable jerking movements, depression, irritability, and dementia. A dramatic effect of basal ganglia malfunction is seen in a condition called hemiballismus. This disorder produces violent, uncontrollable flailing movements of the limbs on one side of the body, which usually subside in 1 to 2 days. Damage to a particular basal ganglia structure – the subthalamic nucleus – on one side of the brain causes hemiballismus, possibly as the result of a minor stroke. Another basal ganglia disorder, known as athetosis, is marked by slow, continual writhing movements.

Where are the basal ganglia?
The basal ganglia include the corpus striatum, the globus pallidus, the substantia nigra, and the subthalamic nucleus. These structures lie below the cortex, deep within the white matter. They control complex patterns of movement, such as walking.

Uncontrollable movements
Normally, the basal ganglia send signals to the cerebral cortex. These signals partially suppress motor commands that move from the motor cortex to the muscles. In Huntington's chorea, parts of the basal ganglia malfunction and the inhibitory influence on the cortex is lost. The result is uncontrollable, jerking movements.

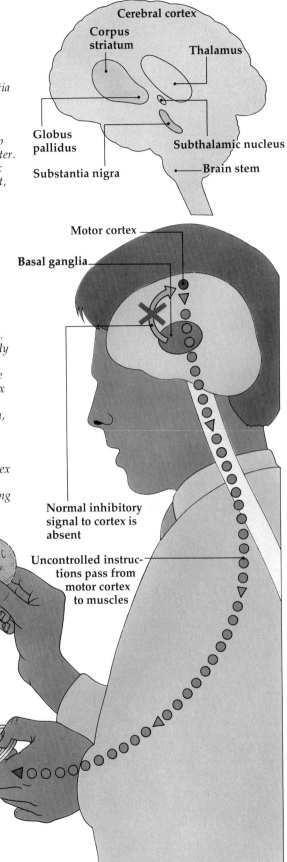

Cerebral cortex
Corpus striatum
Thalamus
Globus pallidus
Substantia nigra
Subthalamic nucleus
Brain stem

Motor cortex
Basal ganglia

Normal inhibitory signal to cortex is absent

Uncontrolled instructions pass from motor cortex to muscles

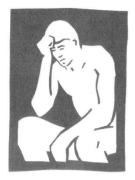

THINKING, UNDERSTANDING, AND KNOWING

THE BRAIN PERCEIVES and interprets information from the senses and then initiates a response. We still don't fully understand how the brain performs these functions. For decades, experts have debated whether the brain functioned as a whole unit or whether separate areas performed distinct tasks. Evidence now suggests that neither view is completely correct.

BEHAVIOR AND EMOTIONS

Our emotions sometimes compel us to take actions that would be morally or socially unacceptable, such as physically hurting a child or crying during a job interview. The human brain is constructed so that we can modify our decisions, actions, and behavior to conform to moral and social laws. This ability to alter our behavior involves the brain's orbitofrontal cortex, part of the frontal lobes, which links decision-making areas (also located in the frontal lobes) with the more primitive limbic system, the seat of feelings and emotions. This ability enables a normal, healthy person to control his or her behavior in a way that is appropriate for a given situation.

Researchers have discovered that certain areas of the brain perform specific functions. They learned this by studying people who sustained injuries that destroyed certain portions of the brain, by stimulating specific areas of the brain with electrical currents and observing the responses, and by using sophisticated imaging techniques to scan brain activity while patients performed various tasks. These methods have targeted the specific brain areas that govern such activities as speaking, moving, and perceiving sensory stimuli.

INTERPRETING AND USING INFORMATION

The areas of the cortex that govern bodily sensation, vision, hearing, and smell perform only a simple analysis of the incoming information. They identify sensations such as delicate touch or coldness, simple visual stimuli such as brightness or color, and aspects of sounds such as loudness or pitch. How we make sense of all this information depends on its further interpretation by the association areas of the cortex.

The association areas of the cortex use stored memories to analyze and compare new information with old. These areas assemble enough data to recognize what this information represents. For example,

When you recognize someone you know
Recognizing someone you know and shouting a greeting seems to be a simple and instantaneous process. But to perform this action, many areas of your brain must interpret complex sensory information and form an appropriate response.

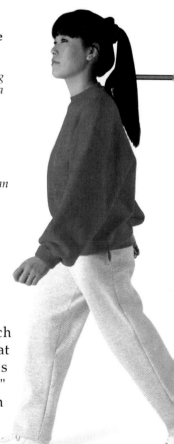

sight and touch may tell you that "this blouse is made of silk." Usually such an analysis happens so fast that you are unaware of the process, but occasionally it proceeds more slowly and becomes conscious, as when you think "I am not sure whether this material is cotton or silk."

The prefrontal cortex puts your thoughts in sequence for use in future planning. It also helps you make decisions, concentrate, and solve problems.

1. Retinas of the eyes
The image of the person is registered by the sensory cells in the retinas of the eyes. These cells respond to color and brightness.

3. Visual association areas of cortex
These areas integrate the individual pieces of information into a complete shape. You first recognize this shape as a human body and then recognize the person.

6. Orbitofrontal cortex
The orbitofrontal cortex and limbic areas recall feelings, such as whether or not you like the person you see.

9. Broca's area
This area plans the words to be spoken and orchestrates the skilled movements needed to articulate these words.

2. Primary visual cortex
The visual signals received by the retinas are relayed to this area. Here, only simple aspects of the visual stimuli are detected, such as borders of images, light and dark contrast, and movement.

4. Angular gyrus
The angular gyrus interprets the meaning of the visual stimulus.

5. Wernicke's area
Wernicke's area converts the visual information into language, associating a name in your mind with the face you see.

7. Prefrontal cortex
The prefrontal cortex puts thoughts into sequence and helps you decide what to do. If you dislike the person, you might ignore him or her; if you like the person, you may call out a greeting.

8. Wernicke's area
If you decide to speak, Wernicke's area forms your thoughts.

10. Motor cortex
The areas of the motor cortex that govern the lips, tongue, and larynx activate the muscles of speech.

11. Muscles of speech
Motor nerve fibers transmit commands to the organs and muscles of speech to produce a shout of greeting.

PROBLEMS OF PERCEPTION AND RECOGNITION

Damage to any of the association areas of the brain, such as from a stroke or tumor, interferes with interpretation of sensory information. This damage causes difficulty in recognizing and identifying the source of the sensory stimuli. A person with damage to visual association areas may not recognize a familiar face – even that of a spouse – although vision is intact. In such cases, recognition occurs when the spouse speaks and the association registers in auditory areas of the brain. Disorders in which sensory perception remains intact but interpretation is impaired are called agnosias, meaning "lack of knowledge."

Recognizing a body part

If part of the brain's "body map" in the sensory cortex (see page 43) becomes damaged, a person may not be able to perceive or recognize a part of his or her own body. Some people who have suffered a stroke in the right parietal lobe of the brain lack recognition of their left arm and leg. If the person's left hand is held up, he or she will identify it as the examiner's hand. Such people have even been known to try to throw a "stranger's leg" out of their bed.

Spatial orientation and attention

Areas of the parietal lobe, particularly on the nondominant side (see page 62), control spatial orientation. The parietal lobe gives us our sense of where we are and how to find our way from one place to another. People with mild malfunction in these areas cannot read maps and get lost while walking in familiar places. People who have severe parietal malfunction, caused by head injury, stroke, or brain tumor, might be unable to navigate across the room, although they may see clearly and walk well.

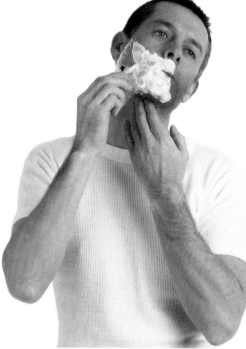

Spatial neglect
A person with damage to certain parts of the parietal cortex may neglect one side of the body when shaving, dressing, or performing other activities. The person may read the print on only one half of a page, may ignore someone talking to him or her from the affected side, and may eat from only one half of his or her plate.

Interpreting visual information
Damage to visual association areas may cause problems interpreting visual information. One example is an inability to separate an object from background images. In a drawing of overlapping images (see right), the person may be able to name one object but not perceive any of the others.

A tumor causing a perceptual disorder
Damage to the somatic sensory association cortex in one hemisphere can result from a tumor. A person affected in this way may be unable to locate a part of his or her body, such as a leg, although he or she is aware of its existence. The person might need help getting dressed.

CASE HISTORY
A PERSONALITY CHANGE

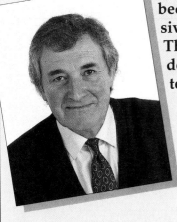

Harold has always **been a popular university lecturer. But recently he became angry at some of his students without provocation. Twice he forgot to attend his lectures. Harold also became uncharacteristically offensive with his colleagues. The concerned head of his department arranged for Harold to see the university psychiatrist.**

PERSONAL DETAILS
Name Harold Bronstein
Age 58
Occupation University professor
Family Harold's parents died of natural causes.

MEDICAL BACKGROUND
Harold has never suffered from a serious disease. He has no personal or family history of a mental disorder and has never abused alcohol or other drugs.

THE PSYCHIATRIC CONSULTATION
When questioned about his health, Harold reports a recent loss of vision in his right eye. Harold appears unconcerned about this symptom and his behavioral changes but mentions that his mood sometimes swings into a deep depression. Considering Harold's reported symptoms, the psychiatrist suspects that Harold may be suffering from damage to the frontal lobe of the brain. The frontal lobes govern thought processes such as concentrating, decision making, and mood and behavior modification. Damage to the frontal lobe would explain Harold's altered personality and recent uncharacteristic behavior. The psychiatrist does not believe Harold has an emotional disorder, so he refers Harold to a neurologist for further tests.

THE NEUROLOGICAL CONSULTATION
While examining Harold's eyes with an ophthalmoscope, the neurologist finds evidence of damage to the right optic nerve. Further tests reveal that Harold has completely lost the sense of smell in his right nostril. These signs, along with Harold's recent uncharacteristic behavior, suggest that something is pressing on Harold's right optic nerve, olfactory tract, and the right frontal lobe tissue lying directly above these structures. The specialist suggests that Harold be scheduled for magnetic resonance imaging of his brain.

THE DIAGNOSIS
The doctors discover that Harold has a TUMOR near the inner surface of his skull, below the right frontal lobe and near the olfactory tract. The tumor is causing Harold's symptoms, including loss of smell, decreased vision, and personality change.

THE TREATMENT
A neurosurgeon removes the growth, which is called a meningioma, a benign tumor that commonly develops from the meninges in this region. The surgery relieves the pressure on Harold's right frontal lobe.

THE OUTCOME
After he is discharged from the hospital, Harold's behavior returns to normal. He resumes his university career but remains partially blind in his right eye from permanent optic nerve damage.

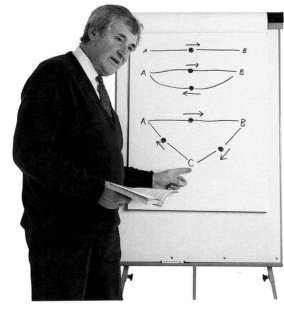

Returning to work
With the tumor removed, Harold's recovery is nearly complete. His behavior, personality, and abilities gradually return to normal. The loss of sight in his right eye is the only permanent effect.

HOW WE COMMUNICATE

Our ability to speak and write sets us apart from lower animals. Our language function is located on one side of the brain. The side of the brain that contains the language function is called the "dominant hemisphere." In natural right-handers, this area is almost always the left side of the brain. In about two thirds of left-handers, the left side is also dominant. In left-handers, dominance for language is not as strongly localized on one side of the brain as in right-handers. This improves the outlook for recovery of speech loss in left-handers who suffer stroke or head injury. Brain hemisphere

A PROBLEM UNDERSTANDING SPEECH

Damage to Wernicke's area causes receptive aphasia, which means difficulty comprehending the meaning of speech sounds. An affected person also cannot monitor his or her own speech output. The person can produce a free flow of speech without difficulty, but it makes little sense.

HEARING AND SPEAKING

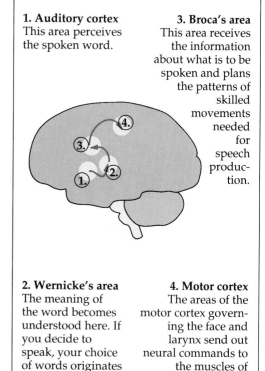

1. Auditory cortex
This area perceives the spoken word.

3. Broca's area
This area receives the information about what is to be spoken and plans the patterns of skilled movements needed for speech production.

2. Wernicke's area
The meaning of the word becomes understood here. If you decide to speak, your choice of words originates in this area.

4. Motor cortex
The areas of the motor cortex governing the face and larynx send out neural commands to the muscles of speech.

READING AND WRITING DIFFICULTIES

Children with dyslexia have difficulty learning to read, spell, and write. Dyslexia may occur in retarded children or can appear as an isolated disability in normal children. In its isolated form, dyslexia more commonly affects left-handed children and occurs more frequently in boys than in girls. Its cause is unknown but may involve incomplete location of language functions in one hemisphere. There may be abnormalities in the language areas. The intellectual abilities of dyslexic children may be normal. Many have an above-average aptitude for art, music, sports, or dancing.

READING AND WRITING

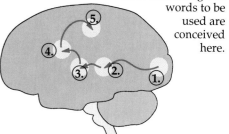

1. Primary visual and visual association areas
These areas perceive the sight of a word.

3. Wernicke's area
The full meaning of the written word is understood here. If you decide to write something, the words to be used are conceived here.

2. Angular gyrus
The early stages of word interpretation occur here. The visual stimulus is also converted here into its linguistic meaning.

4. Broca's area
This area arranges the sequence of movements needed for writing.

5. Motor cortex
From here, neural commands are sent to the muscles involved in writing.

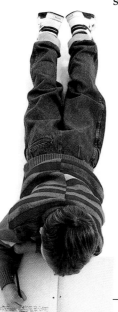

Acquired reading difficulties
Interpretation of visual data occurs in the angular gyrus. Damage to this area makes the person unable to interpret writing, a disorder called acquired alexia. After a stroke or head injury, alexia is usually accompanied by the inability to write (agraphia). People with damage in visual association areas can write, but cannot read what they have written.

Dyslexic children
Dyslexic children occasionally read words from right to left rather than left to right, confusing words like "was" and "saw." Some also have difficulties identifying letters that look similar, such as p, b, q, and d. These problems cause mistakes in the children's writing as well. Non-dyslexic children make such errors when they are learning to read and write but quickly outgrow them.

LEFT- AND RIGHT-HANDEDNESS

Language function seems to be more strictly confined to one side of the brain in right-handed people than in left-handed people. Motor activities are similarly more localized. Right-handed people make up about 89 percent of the population. The remaining 11 percent are left-handed.

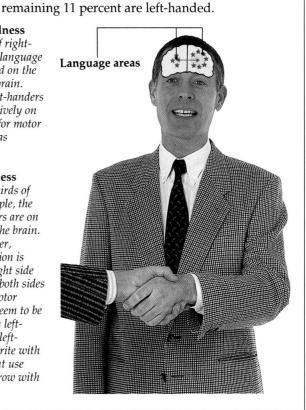

Language area

Language areas

Right-handedness
In 99 percent of right-handed people, language areas are located on the left side of the brain. Almost all right-handers also rely exclusively on the right hand for motor activities such as writing.

Left-handedness
In about two thirds of left-handed people, the language centers are on the left side of the brain. Of the remainder, language function is either on the right side or is shared by both sides of the brain. Motor activities also seem to be less localized in left-handers. Some left-handers may write with the left hand but use scissors and throw with the right hand.

dominance for language is usually well established in children by age 5. If irreversible damage occurs on one side of the brain before that time, the other side can assume language functions.

Areas of the brain involved in language function include Wernicke's area, Broca's area, the angular gyrus, the supramarginal gyrus, the primary visual and visual association areas, and the fibers that connect them. When damage occurs in these areas, the resulting impairment affects both writing and speech and is called aphasia. Aphasia refers to the loss of previously acquired language functions. This means that a retarded child who never learned to speak would not be classified as aphasic. Aphasia can also affect the person's ability to read and comprehend language. The specific symptoms displayed by the person depend on the area of brain damaged.

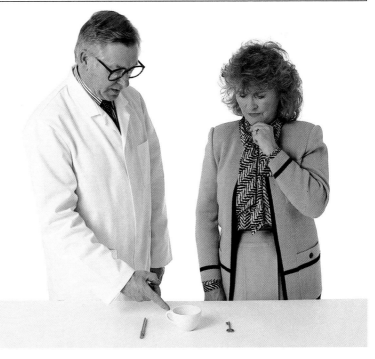

Difficulty naming objects
People with anomic aphasia have lost their memory for words and have difficulty naming objects. Language comprehension is not affected.

THE TWO HEMISPHERES

In most people, the left side of the brain is dominant and controls language function. The same side also governs mathematics skills. The nondominant hemisphere, usually the right hemisphere, regulates spatial orientation. People with damage to the nondominant hemisphere lose their sense of direction, cannot copy simple drawings, and cannot dress themselves properly.

Many human abilities are not strictly localized on one side of the brain. Musical ability seems to involve both hemispheres, although certain aspects of this ability may be localized. Some medical experts consider creativity a nondominant hemispheric function, but creative ability probably requires the coordinated interplay of both hemispheres. Evidence suggests that speech itself, the classic example of a localized function, is partially influenced by the nondominant side of the brain. People with damage to the nondominant side of the brain may lose the usual rhythm and inflection of their speech and cannot interpret these characteristics in the speech of others.

INTELLIGENCE

Despite many attempts to define intelligence, its exact description remains elusive. Intelligence measures a person's ability to comprehend his or her environment, evaluate it rationally, and form

HOW BRAIN FUNCTIONS BECOME LOCALIZED

In over half of newborn babies, Wernicke's area is larger in the left hemisphere than in the right. Because of this, the left Wernicke's area becomes activated more often than the right. This tendency favors the left cerebral hemisphere, which develops rapidly and becomes the dominant side of the brain.

DOMINANT AND NONDOMINANT FUNCTIONS

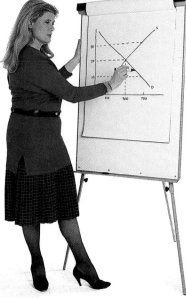

Left hemisphere   **Right hemisphere**

Left Wernicke's area
This area interprets sensory information that can be understood verbally.

Right Wernicke's area
This area interprets patterns of sensory information, such as music, that do not convert into verbal symbols.

The "intuitive" nondominant side
The nondominant hemisphere is important in sensory perception and helps us conceptualize spatial and temporal relationships. It interprets visual and sound patterns, especially in music. This hemisphere may also help us understand nonverbal communication and think intuitively.

The "logical" dominant side
The dominant hemisphere is more involved in rational, verbal, and analytical thinking and logical reasoning. It also performs the sequential analysis needed for mathematical calculations.

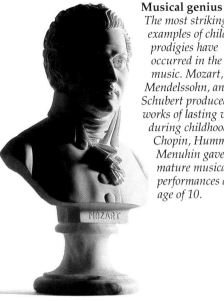

Musical genius
The most striking examples of child prodigies have occurred in the field of music. Mozart, Mendelssohn, and Schubert produced works of lasting value during childhood. Chopin, Hummel, and Menuhin gave mature musical performances at the age of 10.

creative, effective responses to it. Intelligence also defines a person's ability to understand abstract concepts, to reason, and to see the similarities and differences between things. Research shows that intelligence is partly hereditary and partly the product of environment.

Intelligence and education
Some social scientists have pointed out that our current methods of measuring intelligence may be influenced by socioeconomic and other factors. Many psychologists and educators encourage a broader definition of intelligence that also takes into account areas of human ability other than intellect, such as musical, artistic, and physical coordination abilities (usually classified as talents) as well as interpersonal (social) skills and self-understanding. A balanced development of all these abilities best prepares a person for life's many challenges.

In some elementary education programs, children who are poor at mathematics or language skills are given special encouragement in areas – such as music, art, and dance – in which they have exceptional talent. Many of these children develop increased self-confidence that motivates them to try harder and perform better in traditional subjects.

Gifted children
There has always been great interest in child prodigies and other gifted children. In some cases of exceptional ability, the "genius" is limited to a single field of endeavor, such as music. Many gifted individuals have multiple talents.

Research shows that gifted children share some common traits. The first is high intelligence, usually measured by IQ (intelligence quotient) tests. Second, gifted children display abundant creativity, which gives them the ability to solve problems in new or unusual ways. Finally, such children often possess a high motivation to learn, expressed as delight in the pursuit of knowledge. Their talents often lie in such diverse areas as language, mathematics, music, chess, or visual/spatial abilities. Rare instances occur in which a child will display astonishing abilities in one area, such as the ability to play musical pieces on the piano after hearing them only once. How these gifts develop and their location in specific brain areas remain unknown.

HOW DO WE MEASURE INTELLIGENCE?
In 1905, French physiologist Alfred Binet (1857-1911) developed the first intelligence test to gauge the mental abilities of children by comparing them to other children of the same age. By 1916, other experts had developed a formula that found a person's intelligence quotient (IQ). Today many experts believe IQ tests measure only a small part of human intelligence because many people with average IQs excel in life, while some of those with high IQs do not attain success.

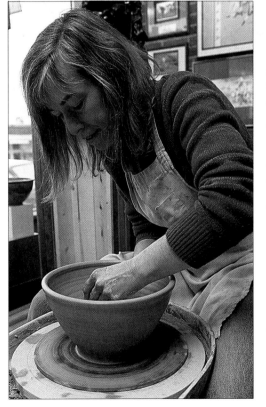

Artistic talent
Several areas of the brain must work together to produce a work of art. Visual artists, such as painters and sculptors, possess great visual/spatial skill in perceiving the world accurately and then representing what they see. Artists also display a vivid imagination and ample creativity in solving problems, such as how to design and construct a building or what to paint on a blank canvas. An artist's rich appreciation of beauty involves his or her emotions. Such all-encompassing ability relies on the integrated functioning of the whole brain.

LEARNING AND MEMORY

When you learn something, such as a foreign language, and then recall it, you engage in a process having three stages. First, registration occurs – you become aware of what needs to be learned. Second, you store the registered information in your memory. This step is called acquisition. Evidence suggests that you enter data into short-term storage and then transfer some of it to long-term memory. Finally, you recall the acquired information later in an act known as retrieval. During this stage, you bring the information stored at an unconscious level into your conscious mind. Many factors determine how well you will remember something, including the amount of attention you give to the subject during the first two stages.

There are several kinds of memory. One kind helps you remember where you left your keys, another kind accumulates your lifelong experience and knowledge, and a third kind helps you remember how to drive a car or ride a bicycle. Each type of memory involves different areas of your brain.

THE STAGES OF MEMORY STORAGE

Brief retention by the brain
Following a sensory experience, the brain can retain the neural signals for only a very short time (several hundred milliseconds). This briefly retained information (the sensory memory) can be scanned to pick out important points.

The temporary memory store
The short-term memory holds information that is currently in use, such as telephone numbers just read from the telephone book. The short-term memory storage capability is quite limited. Most of us can briefly remember a string of eight letters or numbers but not 12. New incoming data permanently displace the contents of the memory store.

Permanent storage
Long-term memory stores information that can be recalled at a later date – from hours to days, months, or years later. The formation of long-term memory involves the transfer of information (called consolidation) from the short-term to the long-term memory stores. Disruption of brain function, such as that from a convulsion or general anesthesia, can prevent the process from occurring.

HOW YOUR BRAIN FORMS MEMORIES

The true nature of the long-term memory remains unknown. Some experts believe that previously inactive genetic material (DNA) "turns on" in the nerve cells involved in memory formation. This process causes the nerve cells to form new types of protein molecules. Such proteins would be needed to bring about the permanent changes that are thought to occur in the nerve cells when a memory is formed.

The hippocampus
In this cross-section of the brain, the hippocampus looks something like a small sea horse, the Greek origin of its name.

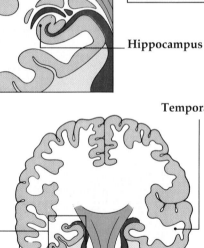

Hippocampus

Temporal lobe

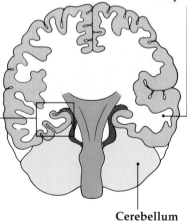

Cerebellum

Selecting what is to be stored
The brain does not store all of the information it receives as memories. The hippocampus, located on the inner border of the temporal lobe, decides which information is important enough to be stored. The information that is selected for storage is usually data that are new and interesting, especially when linked to a strong emotion.

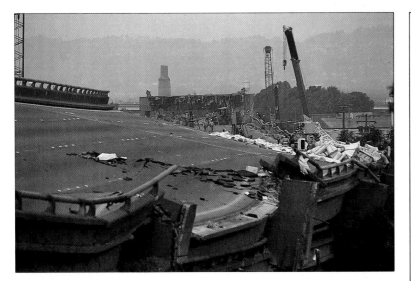

Vivid memories
Details of personal experiences that are highly emotionally charged – such as stressful, exciting, or life-threatening situations – register vividly and accumulate quickly in your memory stores.

HOW TO IMPROVE YOUR MEMORY

How well you remember something depends on how well you stored (learned) it in the first place. Your long-term memory store relies heavily on meaning, organization, order, and association. The better you organize the initial storage process, the more accessible the information – like any other filing system. Verbal and visual links to already-stored information help reinforce the memory processes. The following steps can help you to improve your memory:

◆ Reduce stress by learning relaxation techniques.
◆ Maintain a positive attitude and improve your self-confidence.
◆ Improve your language ability; a good command of language enhances memory.
◆ Repeat to yourself what you wish to learn; try chanting or singing the information, as many children do.
◆ Use visual and verbal mnemonics or memory aids. One type of visual mnemonic associates items on a list with images in a visual scene; remembering the scene helps you to recall the list. An example of a well-known verbal mnemonic is "Every Good Boy Does Fine" for remembering the positions of notes in the treble clef.

MEMORY IMPAIRMENT

The ability to form new memories can be disturbed by lack of concentration, which may arise from depression, anxiety, or a simple lack of interest. Difficulty with recall may follow:

◆ A head injury
◆ Excessive alcohol consumption
◆ Seizure activity in the brain
◆ Electric shock
◆ Tranquilizing drugs, such as diazepam
◆ Dementia, particularly Alzheimer's disease
◆ Obstructed circulation in the brain
◆ Decreased blood flow to the brain following stroke or heart attack
◆ Amnesia caused by shock, such as bereavement

Those brain areas that are crucial to normal memory function include deep portions of the temporal lobes and parts of the thalamus. Many other areas also participate, depending partly on the type of information to be learned. The act of remembering a word, for instance, requires the dominant side of the brain. You learn some nonverbal information with the aid of the nondominant hemisphere. Your brain also learns things such as how to walk or swing a baseball bat – activities that are not usually considered memories. Storage and retrieval of the motor skills needed to perform such tasks engage still other areas of the brain, such as the basal ganglia, the cerebellum, and the cortex of the frontal lobes.

Memory function and age

Many people feel that they are not as mentally sharp in middle age as when they were younger. But studies comparing people with similar educational backgrounds and following groups of individuals over many years have proven that very little loss of memory function occurs before age 70. Before that time, forgetfulness is usually caused by anxiety, fatigue, or stress.

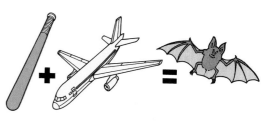

Memory aid
Someone trying to remember to take a baseball bat to the airport when going on vacation might visualize the animal type of bat (a visual image of the same name, also associated with flying) as a memory aid.

CHAPTER THREE

THE UNCONSCIOUS BRAIN

ENCLOSED WITHIN the parts of your brain that govern conscious activity – principally the outer layers of the cerebrum – are many regions that control unconscious functions. These regions work with little or no control by the higher brain centers. They include regions in the center of the brain, such as the hypothalamus and other parts of the limbic system; the pituitary and pineal glands; and parts of the brain stem and its connections to the autonomic (literally "self-governing") nervous system. These regions form the most primitive parts of your brain in terms of evolutionary development. In fact, the unconscious, primitive parts of your human brain differ very little from those of other mammals. The unconscious brain is vitally important to humans. All the functions of your body, such as your breathing, digestive process,

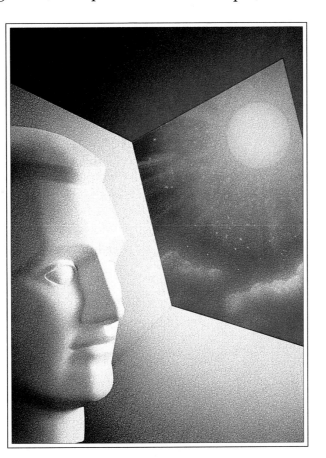

heart rate, body temperature, and blood pressure, are controlled by the unconscious brain. So are the actions of your body's hormonal system. The brain receives signals about your body's internal state and adjusts its functions without your conscious awareness. The unconscious brain also governs instinctive reactions, such as anger and fear, and cyclical behavior patterns, such as sleep. This explains why we sometimes experience apparently irrational reactions to circumstances, for example a fear of heights, and explains why we suffer jet lag when our bodies have to adapt to a time change. Instincts and cyclical behaviors are present in both humans and lower animals. Your cerebral cortex can modify instinctive reactions, but the primitive drives still exist. For example, learned behavior in the cortex modifies the instinct to mate so that we perform this activity only in appropriate circumstances. Your learned behavior can even change the cyclical behavior patterns that govern sleep and eating. Shift workers can adapt to working at night because they can readjust their daily rhythms to a different cycle.

The various regions of your unconscious brain also control actions that you perform automatically. This explains why you can carry out a complex action that you have learned how to do well such as driving a car, while you are thinking about a conversation you had with your boss. The unconscious brain is also responsible for the automatic actions performed during states such as hypnosis and sleep walking. To carry out these automatic activities, the unconscious brain somehow activates learned motor programs and other memories.

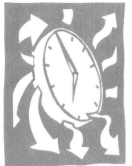

HORMONES AND VITAL FUNCTIONS

YOUR BODY'S vital functions, such as temperature regulation, heart rate, breathing, digestion, and blood pressure, work independently of your conscious control. Two important areas within your brain – the hypothalamus and the brain stem – regulate these automatic functions in your body.

The brain controls your body's involuntary internal processes through two crucial mechanisms: the hormonal system and the nervous system. The hypothalamus, a small, cherry-sized region near the base of the brain that lies just above the pituitary gland, governs the hormonal system through its stimulating and inhibiting influence on the pituitary gland and the hormones this gland secretes. Nervous system control is directed through the activity of the autonomic nervous system.

THE HYPOTHALAMUS

The hypothalamus controls the autonomic nervous system (see page 70) and regulates body temperature (below) and the release of hormones by the pituitary gland (right). Other functions under its complete or partial control include heart rate; blood pressure; regulation of sleep, sexual behavior, and emotion; and food and water intake (see INSTINCTS, CYCLES, AND BEHAVIOR on page 75).

TEMPERATURE REGULATION

The hypothalamus acts like a thermostat. In response to a change in blood temperature, your hypothalamus turns on or off a variety of temperature-regulating mechanisms.

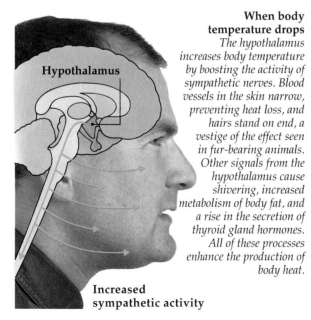

Hypothalamus

When body temperature drops
The hypothalamus increases body temperature by boosting the activity of sympathetic nerves. Blood vessels in the skin narrow, preventing heat loss, and hairs stand on end, a vestige of the effect seen in fur-bearing animals. Other signals from the hypothalamus cause shivering, increased metabolism of body fat, and a rise in the secretion of thyroid gland hormones. All of these processes enhance the production of body heat.

Increased sympathetic activity

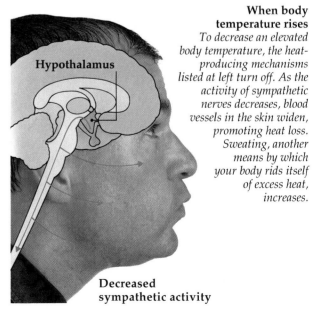

Hypothalamus

When body temperature rises
To decrease an elevated body temperature, the heat-producing mechanisms listed at left turn off. As the activity of sympathetic nerves decreases, blood vessels in the skin widen, promoting heat loss. Sweating, another means by which your body rids itself of excess heat, increases.

Decreased sympathetic activity

HORMONAL CONTROL BY THE BRAIN

The hypothalamus orchestrates the body's endocrine (hormonal) system. Special blood vessels carry hormones from the hypothalamus to the front (anterior) part of the pituitary gland. These hormones trigger the secretion of six other hormones by the front part of the pituitary gland. The back (posterior) part of the pituitary gland, composed of a collection of nerve endings that originate in the hypothalamus, releases three additional hormones. The secretion of many hormones is cyclical.

Hypothalamus

Anterior (front) pituitary gland

Posterior (back) pituitary gland

Releasing hormones

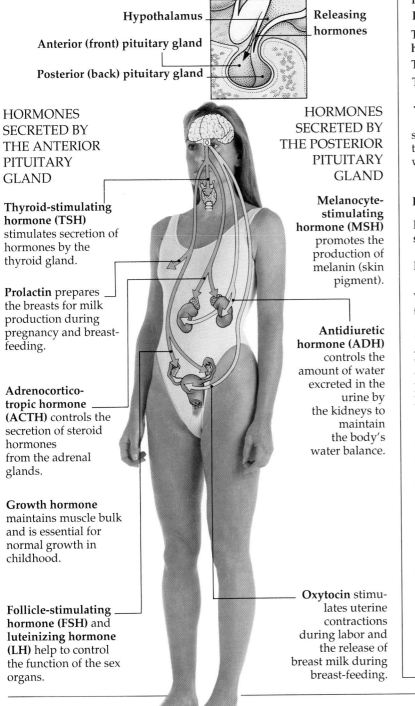

HORMONES SECRETED BY THE ANTERIOR PITUITARY GLAND

Thyroid-stimulating hormone (TSH) stimulates secretion of hormones by the thyroid gland.

Prolactin prepares the breasts for milk production during pregnancy and breast-feeding.

Adrenocortico-tropic hormone (ACTH) controls the secretion of steroid hormones from the adrenal glands.

Growth hormone maintains muscle bulk and is essential for normal growth in childhood.

Follicle-stimulating hormone (FSH) and **luteinizing hormone (LH)** help to control the function of the sex organs.

HORMONES SECRETED BY THE POSTERIOR PITUITARY GLAND

Melanocyte-stimulating hormone (MSH) promotes the production of melanin (skin pigment).

Antidiuretic hormone (ADH) controls the amount of water excreted in the urine by the kidneys to maintain the body's water balance.

Oxytocin stimulates uterine contractions during labor and the release of breast milk during breast-feeding.

FEEDBACK MECHANISMS

Feedback mechanisms operate between a target gland, the hypothalamus, and the pituitary gland to help control hormone production. This is how the process works to regulate the release of thyroid hormone.

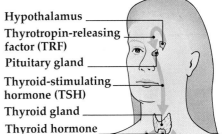

Hypothalamus
Thyrotropin-releasing factor (TRF)
Pituitary gland
Thyroid-stimulating hormone (TSH)
Thyroid gland
Thyroid hormone

1 A hypothalamic hormone, called thyrotropin-releasing factor (TRF), stimulates the pituitary gland to release thyroid-stimulating hormone (TSH), which stimulates the thyroid gland.

Reduced TRF secretion

Reduced TSH secretion

Negative feedback

Too much thyroid hormone

2 If thyroid hormone levels rise too high, feedback mechanisms stimulate the hypothalamus to reduce TRF production. The secretion of TSH and thyroid hormone drops, which reduces hormonal levels to normal.

Increased TRF secretion

Increased TSH secretion

Weakened feedback

Too little thyroid hormone

3 If thyroid hormone levels drop, the feedback weakens and the hypothalamus increases its production of TRF. This factor stimulates TSH and thyroid hormone production, which returns levels to normal.

AUTONOMIC NERVOUS SYSTEM

The autonomic nervous system has two divisions: the sympathetic and para-sympathetic. Sympathetic nervous system activity predominates during times of stress, while parasympathetic activity prevails during rest and recuperation. The nerve fibers of these two divisions leave the brain and spinal cord by way of the cranial and spinal nerves, respectively, to supply organs and other internal structures. The drawings on these two pages illustrate the actions and effects of the sympathetic and parasympathetic nervous systems. Not all organs interact with both systems; blood vessels, for example, are supplied only by sympathetic nerves.

EFFECTS OF PARASYMPATHETIC NERVE ACTIVITY

The parasympathetic nervous system promotes and regulates processes such as digestion and growth. By allowing the body to rest and recuperate, its activities save energy.

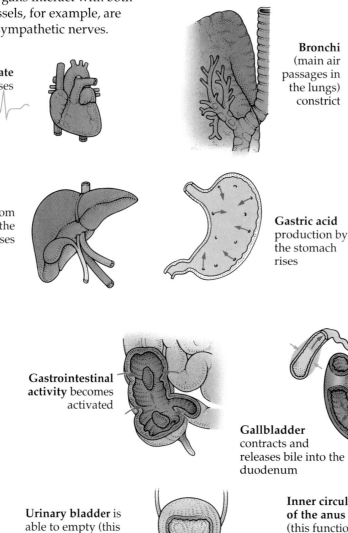

Pupils constrict

Saliva production by the salivary glands increases

Bronchi (main air passages in the lungs) constrict

Gastric acid production by the stomach rises

Gallbladder contracts and releases bile into the duodenum

Inner circular muscle of the anus relaxes (this function is partially under conscious control in adults)

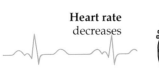

Heart rate decreases

Glucose release from the liver into the bloodstream ceases

Gastrointestinal activity becomes activated

Urinary bladder is able to empty (this function is partially under conscious control in adults)

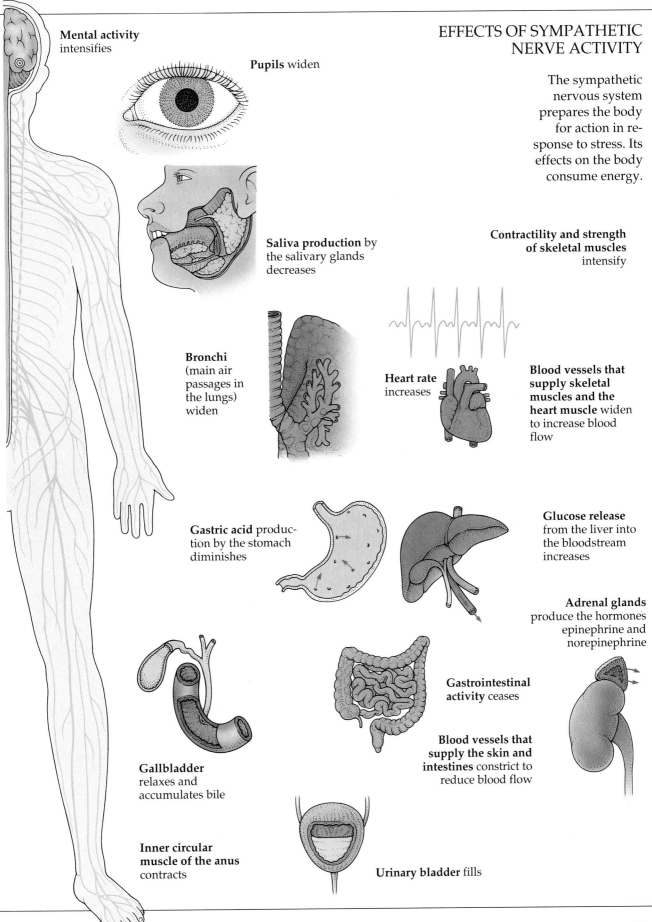

Mental activity intensifies

Pupils widen

EFFECTS OF SYMPATHETIC NERVE ACTIVITY

The sympathetic nervous system prepares the body for action in response to stress. Its effects on the body consume energy.

Saliva production by the salivary glands decreases

Contractility and strength of skeletal muscles intensify

Bronchi (main air passages in the lungs) widen

Heart rate increases

Blood vessels that supply skeletal muscles and the heart muscle widen to increase blood flow

Gastric acid production by the stomach diminishes

Glucose release from the liver into the bloodstream increases

Adrenal glands produce the hormones epinephrine and norepinephrine

Gastrointestinal activity ceases

Gallbladder relaxes and accumulates bile

Blood vessels that supply the skin and intestines constrict to reduce blood flow

Inner circular muscle of the anus contracts

Urinary bladder fills

THE BRAIN STEM

The brain stem is the lowest section of the brain. The brain stem helps control coordinated eye movements, facial movement and sensation, hearing, and swallowing. It also serves as a pathway for messages traveling between other parts of the brain and the spinal cord. Finally, the brain stem contains vital centers involved in the control of your heart rate, breathing, blood pressure, and sleep/wake cycles. The brain stem consists of three parts, called the midbrain, pons, and medulla.

ESSENTIAL HYPERTENSION

For reasons not fully understood, many people develop persistently elevated blood pressure during middle age. People with high blood pressure are at increased risk of heart attack and stroke. These risks can be reduced by treatment with drugs that lower blood pressure.

Control of heart rate

Cardiac centers in the medulla, which can alter sympathetic and parasympathetic activity, assume primary control of your heart rate. When you are faced with a stressful situation, your heart rate increases. This happens because your cardiac centers arouse sympathetic nerves, which in turn stimulate the heart directly. During stress, your adrenal glands also release two hormones – norepinephrine and epinephrine – which stimulate your heart to beat faster.

The cardiac centers receive information from other parts of the brain and body that helps them determine how to control heart rate. One factor that influences the cardiac centers to boost heart rate is the detection of reduced blood pressure by pressure receptors in arteries. Others include signals from the cerebral cortex and limbic system that indicate excitement and anger, signals of extreme pain, detection of blood chemical changes caused by exercise, and signals from stretch receptors in the lungs that indicate inhalation.

Control of breathing

The medulla contains a respiratory center, modified by input from higher regions in the brain stem, that controls your breathing rate. This respiratory center stimulates the phrenic nerves that supply the diaphragm (the horizontal muscle that separates the chest from the abdomen) and the intercostal nerves that supply the chest wall muscles. Increased carbon dioxide levels in the blood prompt the respiratory center to act. As breathing increases, the bloodstream absorbs more oxygen from the lungs, while carbon dioxide is flushed out.

The respiratory center sends signals to increase breathing and stimulates the cardiac centers to increase heart rate simultaneously. Control of breathing and heart rate are closely linked and the control centers for each of these functions lie close to each other.

BLOOD PRESSURE CONTROL

In healthy people, the bodily mechanisms that control blood pressure operate continuously to maintain blood pressure at an optimum level. Sensory pressure receptors in the aorta (the large artery that carries blood from the heart) and in the carotid arteries of the neck constantly monitor your blood pressure so it does not rise too high or fall too low. Nerves transmit this information to vital cardiac centers in the medulla, which affect the width of blood vessels and the heart rate.

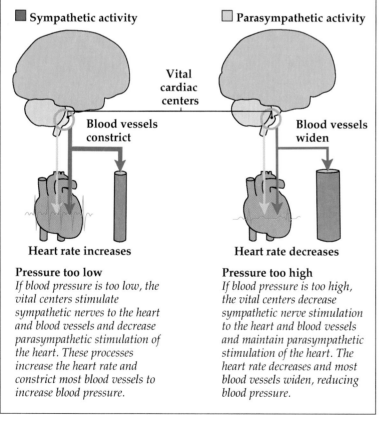

■ **Symphathetic activity** □ **Parasympathetic activity**

Vital cardiac centers

Blood vessels constrict

Blood vessels widen

Heart rate increases **Heart rate decreases**

Pressure too low
If blood pressure is too low, the vital centers stimulate sympathetic nerves to the heart and blood vessels and decrease parasympathetic stimulation of the heart. These processes increase the heart rate and constrict most blood vessels to increase blood pressure.

Pressure too high
If blood pressure is too high, the vital centers decrease sympathetic nerve stimulation to the heart and blood vessels and maintain parasympathetic stimulation of the heart. The heart rate decreases and most blood vessels widen, reducing blood pressure.

CASE HISTORY
A PERSISTENT FEELING OF FULLNESS

OLIVIA RECENTLY had been suffering from an uncomfortable feeling of fullness that began during meals and persisted afterward. Her son took her to an expensive restaurant and was surprised when she complained about discomfort and was unable to finish her meal. He urged his mother to see her doctor.

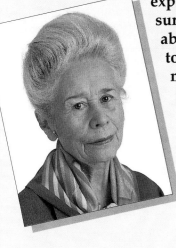

PERSONAL DETAILS
Name Olivia Watson
Age 64
Occupation Office manager
Family No history of gastrointestinal disease.

MEDICAL BACKGROUND

Olivia was told she had maturity-onset diabetes mellitus 10 years ago. She was initially given medication and placed on a special diet. Recently, she has allowed her treatment to lapse. She has also neglected medical checkups and has not had her blood checked or her urine tested for sugar.

THE CONSULTATION

The doctor examines Olivia's abdomen and finds no obvious abnormalities. But he detects evidence in the retinas of Olivia's eyes of uncontrolled diabetes. He suspects that her diabetes has been uncontrolled for some time, so he orders several tests to determine its extent.

THE INVESTIGATIONS

Olivia's blood sugar level is elevated, and her glycosylated hemoglobin level (a change in the red blood cell pigment caused by a reaction with glucose) is very high. These results confirm the doctor's suspicions about Olivia's diabetes, which prompt him to investigate Olivia's stomach problems. Olivia is asked to swallow a special liquid that will highlight her gastrointestinal organs on X-rays. The X-rays reveal that Olivia suffers from delayed gastric emptying, which means the passage of food from her stomach to her small intestine is delayed.

THE DIAGNOSIS

The doctor tells Olivia that she has DIABETIC GASTROPARESIS, a nerve degeneration that affects the parasympathetic nerves supplying her stomach and the sympathetic nerves supplying the circular muscles leading from her stomach. These nerves regulate normal gastric function. Their degeneration causes delayed emptying of the stomach contents after a meal, resulting in the feeling of fullness.

THE TREATMENT

A strict diabetic diet lowers Olivia's blood sugar levels to normal. Her gastric symptoms do not improve, because the nerve damage is irreversible. But the doctor prescribes a drug called metoclopramide to speed gastric emptying.

THE OUTCOME

After Olivia begins taking her medication, most of her symptoms subside, and her appetite returns. She resolves to maintain good diabetic control and to stick rigidly to her diet. Five years later, her diabetes is well controlled, and the gastroparesis has not worsened.

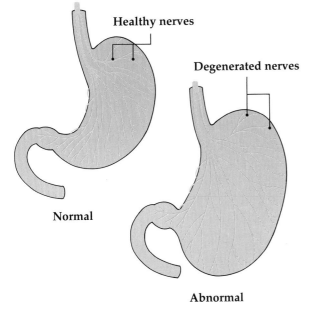

Healthy nerves

Degenerated nerves

Normal

Abnormal

The root of the problem
The doctor explains to Olivia that her symptoms result from delayed gastric emptying. The nerve supply to the stomach and to the muscles leading from it, which normally promotes digestion, has degenerated, causing Olivia's condition. Because the stomach is not emptying normally, it becomes distended, as shown in the illustration at left.

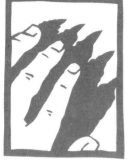

INSTINCTS, CYCLES, AND BEHAVIOR

SCIENTISTS HAVE LONG studied the processes that regulate animal behavior. All animals have instincts. They are biologically programmed to respond in a certain way when faced with specific environmental conditions or internal cues. Instinct moves birds to build nests and spiders to weave webs. Human instinct is most evident in such behavior patterns as the sleep/wake cycle.

In the early 1900s, scientists believed that human behavior was controlled by instinct. Today, scientists reserve instinctive theories of behavior for lower animals in which complex behaviors are programmed genetically and exhibited even when an animal has never been in contact with another member of its species. Humans exhibit innate behaviors, such as sucking, particularly in infancy.

LIMBIC SYSTEM CONTROL OF INSTINCTS

Instinctive behavior, controlled by the limbic system, protects us from environmental hazards and ensures survival. In humans, the limbic system is linked to the higher parts of the cortex, allowing us to greatly modify our instincts. Here are some examples of differences in animal and human behavior.

The limbic system
Some of the key areas of the limbic system are shown here.

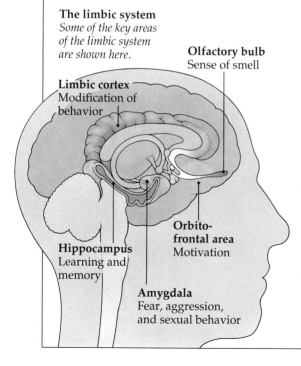

Limbic cortex
Modification of behavior

Olfactory bulb
Sense of smell

Hippocampus
Learning and memory

Orbito-frontal area
Motivation

Amygdala
Fear, aggression, and sexual behavior

Human sexual instincts
Human sexual behavior involves many parts of the nervous system. The urge to copulate is governed by the limbic system but is modulated by the cortex. Information that enters the limbic system, such as the sight of someone you are attracted to, stimulates the autonomic nervous system

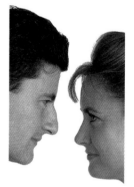

via the hypothalamus and triggers the reflexes that enable copulation to occur. Because learned psychological and social factors modify human sexual behavior, it is much more difficult to define a "normal" range of behavior for humans than for lower animals.

Fear and rage in humans
Fear and rage are protective instincts that are probably derived from the primitive instincts of our early ancestors. When we feel threatened, our first response is fear and we seek to escape. If escape is impossible, rage (one of many forms of aggression) takes control and we fight. This is the so-called fight or flight response. Specific

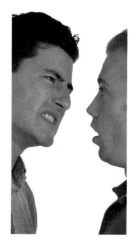

stimuli probably trigger fear or rage, but their nature is unknown. Although humans can largely control fear and rage, men in particular may experience extreme rage due to the effects of the male hormone testosterone on the limbic system. People who suffer from irrational fears and phobias exhibit inappropriate fear responses.

Most human behavior is influenced by learning rather than by instinct. Human sexual instincts, eating behavior, and fear and rage responses can all be modified by thought, arising from the cerebral cortex, in response to learned cues.

NERVOUS SYSTEM CONTROL OF BEHAVIOR

The parts of the brain that are involved in the control of human instincts and cyclical behavior patterns are the limbic system, the hypothalamus, the brain stem, and possibly the pineal gland. In evolutionary terms, the limbic system is the oldest part of the forebrain. Lower mammals possess a highly developed limbic system, which is closely associated

SEXUAL RECOGNITION AND RESPONSE

The limbic system plays a role in sexual recognition and response by receiving and interpreting sights, sounds, odors, and touch sensations. Insects and animals secrete substances called pheromones to arouse a mate's sense of smell. Signals travel through the olfactory bulb into the limbic system, enabling the animal to recognize that a member of the opposite sex is ready to mate. The strength of the pheromone signal varies among species. For example, the female hawk moth secretes pheromones that the male can detect a mile away.

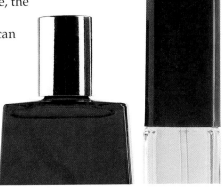

Human pheromones
Pheromones may explain why humans are sexually attracted to some people and not to others. Perfumes often contain the pheromones of animals that may disguise our pheromones.

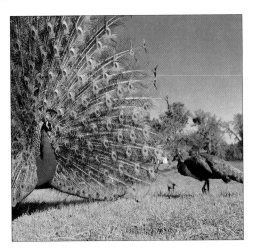

Sexual instincts in lower animals
Lower animals conform to far more rigid patterns of sexual behavior than do humans. For example, some species display elaborate courtship behavior that is biologically programmed. Mating is often confined to a specific season.

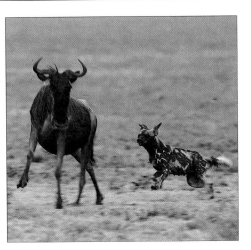

Fear and rage in lower animals
Lower animals exhibit the fight or flight response in the face of danger, but the stimuli that trigger fear and rage are more explicit. The limbic system of each species is programmed to interpret different types of stimuli to produce the appropriate protective response.

with their sense of smell. The neocortex (the part of the cerebral cortex that is separate from the limbic cortex) is most highly developed in humans.

The human limbic system governs emotions, sexual behavior, motivation, sense of smell, and eating. This is why appetite sometimes changes with changing moods. The limbic system brings about bodily changes by stimulating the hypothalamus, which is connected to the body's autonomic nervous system and hormonal system.

The role of emotion

Much human activity is governed by emotions – including hope, enthusiasm, and despair – that have no counterparts in lower animals. The wide range of human emotions that originate in the limbic system reflect the complexity of the human brain's higher functions. No single area within the limbic system controls the full spectrum of emotions.

The limbic system controls mood through connections to the orbitofrontal cortex (see page 56), which regulates motivation. This relationship explains, for example, why motivation is greatly reduced during depression.

BODY RHYTHMS

Many animal activities conform to a variety of cyclical patterns. Such rhythms reflect the 24-hour rotation of the earth on its axis, the monthly rotation of the moon around the earth, or the yearly rotation of the earth around the sun.

Cycles that last approximately 24 hours are known as circadian, a name derived from the Latin words circa, meaning about, and dies, meaning day. The sleep/wake cycle, body temperature, gastric secretion, kidney function, and many other physiological processes follow cyclical circadian rhythms.

Rhythms shorter than 24 hours are known as ultradian. One example is the 90-minute rhythm of dreaming during sleep. Rhythms longer than 24 hours, such as the monthly menstrual cycle, are known as infradian.

Studies of biological rhythms

Research shows that even in caves or windowless apartments that provide no environmental cues, such as sunrise and sunset, biological rhythms continue to influence behavior. These findings suggest that animals have internal regulating mechanisms, called biological clocks. Many studies show that the body's master clock lies in the hypothalamus.

Biological rhythms alter susceptibility to many illnesses. Heart attacks and asthma attacks, for example, are more common in the morning. Signs and symptoms also follow a daily rhythm. Blood pressure, for instance, peaks in late afternoon.

The times of day treatment is given may affect recovery. In one study, survival rates from cancer improved markedly when patients received anticancer drugs at the time calculated to kill the largest number of cancer cells.

Recent research shows that annual rhythms also play an important role in human life. About one in four persons living at middle to northern latitudes reports seasonal changes in mood, sleep, and appetite. An estimated 5 percent of the US population suffers from winter depression. Exposure to artificial lights, at least five times brighter than ordinary room lights, brings relief to many of these people.

CAVE STUDIES

During studies of human biological rhythms, volunteers were deprived of cues that indicate the passage of time, such as variations in light and dark. They could go to sleep and arise at will. Volunteers in these time-free studies almost always followed a daily schedule that was about 25 hours long, which indicates a built-in biological clock in close synchrony with the earth's 24-hour rotation. The natural desire to lengthen the day explains why it is easier to stay up later than to go to bed earlier and why travel in a westward direction is easier than travel eastward.

JET LAG

When crossing time zones, you experience a day that is longer or shorter than the 24-hour period to which your body is accustomed. Travel across time zones can make you sleepy during the day or wakeful at night. You may have gastrointestinal upsets and exhibit poorer performance than usual. These common symptoms, collectively known as jet lag, reflect the effects of altering your body's internal rhythms and interfering with your sleep/wake cycle. At a new destination, you may have to sleep when you would ordinarily be awake and stay up when you would ordinarily sleep. It may take several days to readjust, roughly 1 day for each time zone crossed. Most people experience further disruption after coming home.

Relieving jet lag symptoms
Doctors suggest altering your sleep patterns to relieve jet lag. Try to sleep and eat on local time in the new time zone. Spend time outdoors in the morning when traveling east, in the afternoon when traveling west. It is also a good idea to avoid drinking alcohol.

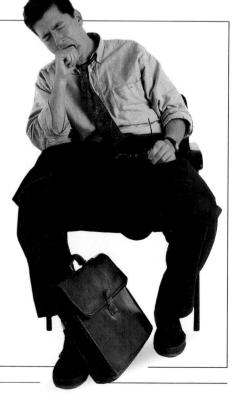

SLEEP DISORDERS

Sleep disorders can involve difficulty falling asleep or staying asleep or trouble staying awake during the day. The causes for these common symptoms may be as diverse as narcolepsy (a neurological disorder), sleep apnea (a respiratory disorder), or jet lag. Sleep disorders also involve events that intrude into sleep or occur during sleep, such as sleep walking and teeth grinding. They may reflect medical or psychiatric disorders, such as epilepsy and depression. The investigation of sleep disorders involves physicians and other specialists in pulmonary medicine, psychiatry, neurology, psychology, pediatrics, and other disciplines. Sleep experts described 84 different sleep disorders in a catalogue published in 1990. The following are some examples:

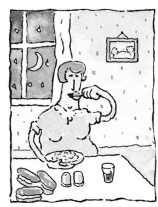 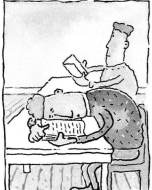 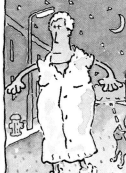 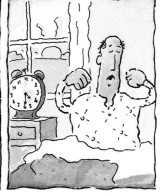

◆ A woman sleeps for 18 hours every day, waking up only to eat and use the bathroom.

◆ A college student can't fall asleep until 3 or 4 AM and sleeps through his morning classes.

◆ An 80-year-old woman gets out of bed during the night and wanders down the street in her nightgown.

◆ A man suffering from depression wakes up early in the morning and can't get back to sleep.

WHAT IS SLEEP?

Sleep is a state during which brain activity differs from that during the waking state. Sleep is an active mental process that does not involve a "turning off" of the brain as scientists once believed. If we were completely unconscious during sleep, we would never hear a crying baby or the siren of a passing fire engine.

Although sleep is a natural state, we knew little about sleep patterns until the sleep studies of the 1960s and 1970s. In these studies, researchers observed healthy volunteers during normal sleep and recorded their brain impulses by electroencephalography (EEG). These studies revealed that we alternate between two different states of sleep known as nonrapid eye movement (NREM) sleep and rapid eye movement (REM) sleep, during which most dreaming takes place. Each type of sleep exhibits different physiological features (see page 78).

Shift work
Shift work, in which people often work at night or alternate between day and night schedules, is on the rise in the US. Some people adapt to shift work easily; most find it difficult. Sleep research shows that people have difficulty adjusting to daytime sleep or varying sleep times. Shift workers usually suffer from sleep deprivation that builds up over time. Lack of sleep may affect work performance. Sleep experts note that many major industrial accidents have occurred at night, when workers who monitored equipment were probably not optimally alert.

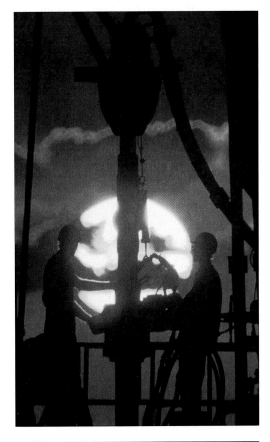

WHAT HAPPENS WHEN YOU SLEEP?

During sleep, we alternate between two different states of sleep every 90 to 100 minutes, as illustrated in the graph below. The first state, known as nonrapid eye movement (NREM) or orthodox sleep, may be divided into four stages of progressively deepening sleep. The second state is known as rapid eye movement (REM) or paradoxical sleep. Patterns produced by recording the brain's electrical activity via electroencephalography (EEG) reflect differences in brain activity during all stages of sleep.

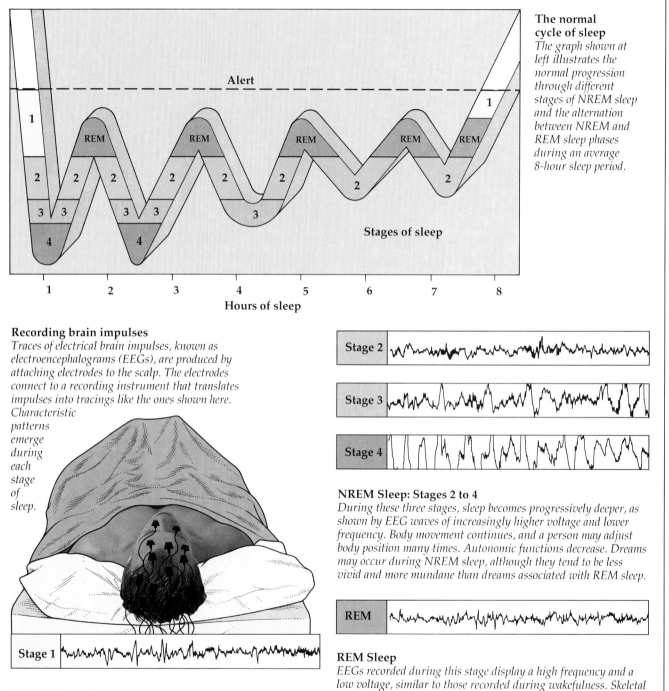

The normal cycle of sleep
The graph shown at left illustrates the normal progression through different stages of NREM sleep and the alternation between NREM and REM sleep phases during an average 8-hour sleep period.

Recording brain impulses
Traces of electrical brain impulses, known as electroencephalograms (EEGs), are produced by attaching electrodes to the scalp. The electrodes connect to a recording instrument that translates impulses into tracings like the ones shown here. Characteristic patterns emerge during each stage of sleep.

Stage 1

NREM Sleep: Stage 1
During this stage, responsiveness to environmental stimuli diminishes and thoughts begin to drift as the body gradually relaxes. NREM stage 1 sleep is a transitional state between wakefulness and sleep.

Stage 2

Stage 3

Stage 4

NREM Sleep: Stages 2 to 4
During these three stages, sleep becomes progressively deeper, as shown by EEG waves of increasingly higher voltage and lower frequency. Body movement continues, and a person may adjust body position many times. Autonomic functions decrease. Dreams may occur during NREM sleep, although they tend to be less vivid and more mundane than dreams associated with REM sleep.

REM

REM Sleep
EEGs recorded during this stage display a high frequency and a low voltage, similar to those recorded during wakefulness. Skeletal muscle movement is inhibited, but the eyes move in all directions, often rapidly. Autonomic functions may increase, as evidenced by more variable breathing and heart rate and by penile erection. Spontaneous ejaculation occasionally occurs in men. Dreams most often occur throughout REM sleep.

DREAM THEORIES

Although some people insist they never dream, people studied in sleep laboratories rarely fail to do so. Whether we need to dream has yet to be established. Some conflicting theories about why we dream appear below:

◆ **The "white noise" theory** Dreams may result from random firing of nerve cells in the reticular activating system during sleep. The brain's struggle to perform its usual task of interpretation may produce dream experiences, but no sensible meaning can be ascribed to them. Thus, dreams have been likened to the white noise produced by a badly tuned radio.

◆ **Dreaming as part of the memory process** Dreams may form part of the process by which short-term memories are committed to long-term storage. When asked to memorize a list of nonsense words and to repeat them 8 and 24 hours later, people remember more words after 24 hours with an intervening period of sleep.

◆ **Dreams as a key to the unconscious** Psychiatrists such as Sigmund Freud and Carl Jung believed that dream analysis could reveal emotional conflicts. Many psychiatrists believe that dreams express these conflicts through images and symbols woven into a story. The dream's meaning must be understood in the context of the person's life and is often revealed during psychoanalysis.

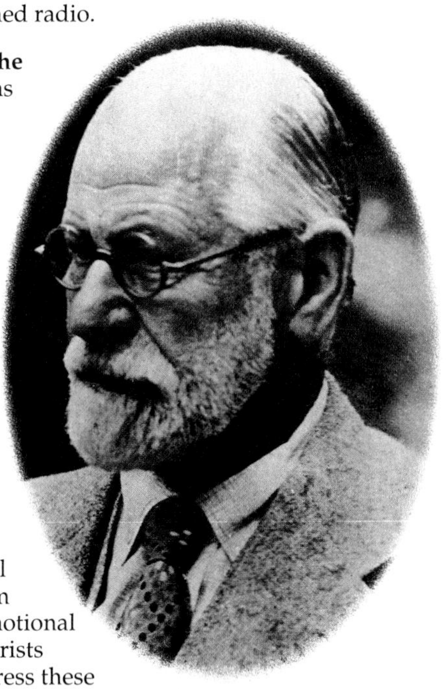

Sigmund Freud (1856-1939)

Why do we sleep?

Sleep deprivation studies have shown that when a person remains awake for unusually long periods, he or she is less able to perform tasks calling for vigilance, such as monitoring a computer screen. But sleep-deprived people can manage tasks calling for physical activity, such as marching, reasonably well. Individuals deprived of sleep for several days become disoriented and occasionally exhibit psychotic symptoms. These and other detrimental effects of sleep deprivation confirm the notion that sleep is vital to human health.

ASK YOUR DOCTOR
SLEEP AND SLEEP DISORDERS

Q My mother, who is in her 70s, claims she never sleeps for more than 3 hours a night and feels fine. Can this be true?

A Yes. Most people need 7 to 8 hours of sleep a night, but some require much less. Sleep often diminishes with age and the elderly are more prone to experience disturbed sleep than are younger people.

Q My husband feels sleepy all day and seems to stop breathing occasionally during the night. What could be wrong?

A Your husband may be suffering from obstructive sleep apnea syndrome, in which breathing can stop for 10 seconds or longer. The problem is diagnosed by monitoring vital functions during sleep. His doctor may be able to control the problem with a treatment called continuous positive airway pressure. Your husband would wear a mask during sleep through which air from an air compressor would flow into his nasal passages to keep them open.

Q Do people who suffer from insomnia actually sleep longer than they realize?

A Research suggests that some insomnia sufferers sleep more than they realize. In some people, the boundaries between wakefulness and sleep become blurred. Although they get 6 to 7 hours of sleep, people with insomnia insist they have slept only a few hours or not at all. One study revealed that insomniacs awakened during the night often failed to realize they had been asleep.

UNDEFINED STATES

D O YOU TAKE the same route to work every day? Once you've established this routine, your mind may begin to wander. You may not even remember portions of the trip. You wouldn't say you've been unconscious. But were you fully conscious? We measure consciousness by degrees. Some states, such as hypnosis and sleepwalking, defy classification.

A person may function without being fully aware of what he or she is doing, a phenomenon called "automatism." Actions performed can range from highly skilled to uncoordinated. Examples of automatism include unconscious actions performed during sleepwalking, in a posthypnotic state, and during or after an epileptic seizure. Some actions performed under normal conditions can also be described as automatisms. Well-developed skills, such as typing or playing a musical instrument, involve highly complex movements that are performed almost automatically.

Learned skills become automatic
Normal automatisms, such as skilled typing, function like a computer program. When you touch the keys, your brain activates a motor memory. The brain sends instructions to the muscles so quickly that your fingers can type automatically, without needing your further conscious direction.

SLEEPWALKING

Researchers once believed that sleepwalkers were acting out their dreams. But electroencephalographic (EEG) recordings, which measure the brain's electrical activity, showed that sleepwalking is most frequently associated with deep, non-dreaming sleep. Sleepwalking occurs most frequently in young children and less frequently as we get older, corresponding to the decline in deep sleep in older adults. We don't know what causes sleepwalking.

The sleepwalker
The sleepwalker – most commonly a young child – seems to be dazed and unaware of his or her surroundings and is somewhat clumsy, yet avoids obstacles. He or she may go through the motions of seemingly purposeful actions, such as sweeping the floor or using the toilet, and may return to bed without help.

HYPNOSIS

Hypnosis is recognized as a distinct state of consciousness. But we don't know much about the way it works. While hypnotized, the subject experiences imaginary sensations or loss of sensation, acts in response to the hypnotist's suggestions, and can even be persuaded to change his or her beliefs. For example, the hypnotist may convince the subject not to hear a particular sound, such as a watch ticking. Under hypnosis, if told that a fly has landed on his or her cheek, the subject may grimace or brush the imagined fly away. Hypnotists' suggestions have even convinced people that they can feel no pain, and doctors have performed apparently pain-free operations on hypnotized patients.

Posthypnotic suggestion

Suggestions made during hypnosis may induce the hypnotized subject to express certain beliefs or perform actions after hypnosis (posthypnotic suggestion). The subject usually then forgets the experience (amnesia). But hypnotized people generally cannot be forced to perform actions they find morally offensive.

Hypnosis has also been used to help people stop or modify unwanted habits, such as smoking and overeating, and to reduce stress. The ability to break habits or addictions can probably be explained by the effects of suggestion combined with the person's lower level of anxiety or self-consciousness about the habit. Some psychotherapists use hypnosis to help their patients remember and cope with repressed events and feelings or to help them relax.

EPILEPTIC AUTOMATISM

This phenomenon occurs after a certain type of psychomotor seizure, affecting areas of the brain within the temporal lobe (see page 94). These actions performed in an epileptic state may be simple movements or complex sequences of behavior but generally are harmless. For example, the person may repeatedly button and unbutton clothing or stack and restack objects.

Hypnosis
Heightened mental awareness, suggestibility, and deep relaxation characterize hypnosis. The subject usually moves into the hypnotic state by concentrating on the hypnotist's voice or by focusing on an object.

Brain waves during hypnosis
EEG recordings of hypnotized subjects' brain waves show waveforms that match those found in subjects who are awake but relaxed, with eyes closed. This finding disproves the theory that hypnotized subjects are asleep.

CHAPTER FOUR

DISORDERS OF THE BRAIN AND NERVOUS SYSTEM

PHYSICAL DISORDERS of the brain and nervous system, called neurological disorders, can cause both physical disability and mental impairment. As researchers find that more and more mental and emotional illnesses can be explained by physical disorders of the brain, such as neurotransmitter imbalances, the distinction between neurological and psychiatric (mental and emotional) disorders is narrowing.

Disorders of the brain and nervous system account for a large percentage of deaths in the US, and they represent an even larger component of overall disability. Many brain and nervous system disorders, such as brain tumors, Huntington's chorea, amyotrophic lateral sclerosis (Lou Gehrig's disease), and trigeminal neuralgia, occur comparatively rarely. Others, such as stroke and serious head injury, are very common. Stroke is responsible for about one tenth of all deaths in the US. After heart disease and cancer, stroke is the third most common cause of death in the US. There are currently almost 1 million people who have survived a stroke, but many are left with some residual physical or mental disability.

Many other nervous system disorders, such as multiple sclerosis, epilepsy, ce-

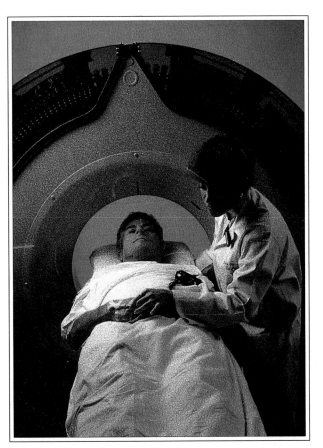

rebral palsy, and Parkinson's disease, also impose a major burden on health care resources and on caregivers. Head injuries incurred in motor-vehicle accidents, sports activities, and assaults are the principal causes of brain and nervous system damage in young adults. Many of these injuries cause permanent paralysis of the arms and legs or lead to mental impairment. Head injuries account for about 1 percent of all deaths in the US. Because of the nervous system's limited capacity for repair, many disorders were considered untreatable until recently. Today, some of the major nervous system disorders successfully respond to medical and neurosurgical treatment. Rehabilitation of people who have disabilities has also improved dramatically. Parkinson's disease, migraine, and epilepsy are often effectively controlled by drug therapy, and many brain and spinal cord tumors and malformations can be removed or corrected.

This chapter begins with an overview of disorders of the brain and nervous system. We explain how new imaging techniques work. Later sections cover some of the most important conditions, such as epilepsy, tumors, head injury, dementia, stroke, and Parkinson's disease.

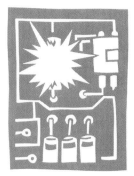

WHAT CAN GO WRONG?

YOUR BRAIN and nervous system have many built-in protective mechanisms. When these mechanisms fail, things can go wrong. Medical science continues to find ways to treat brain and nervous system disorders, although the origins of many of these disorders remain unknown.

Neurologists (doctors who specialize in treating disorders of the brain and nervous system) often categorize disorders according to their underlying cause, such as physical injury or infection. If the exact cause is not known, doctors might categorize the disorder according to its main effects in the brain, such as a neurotransmitter disturbance.

The table on pages 85 and 86 describes the principal categories of brain and nervous system disorders and lists examples of each type. Some disorders fit into more than one category. For exam-

ple, Huntington's chorea can be classified as a genetic disorder, but because this disorder also shows a characteristic lack of the neuro-transmitter gamma-aminobutyric acid (GABA) in certain parts of the brain, it can also be classified as a neurotransmitter disturbance. The exact causes of many serious syndromes and disorders remain unknown or uncertain. They may arise from several different causes. The cause of degenerative disorders, such as Alzheimer's disease and Parkinson's disease, may involve several factors.

Incidence of serious neurological disorders
This graph shows the approximate numbers of new cases of serious neurological disorders that occurred in the US each year in the 1980s per 100,000 people.

Huntington's chorea	0.5
Motor neuron disease	1
Multiple sclerosis	2
Primary brain tumor (arising directly from brain tissue)	10
Parkinson's disease	20
Epilepsy	50
Stroke and other cerebrovascular disease	200

DISORDERS OF THE BRAIN AND NERVOUS SYSTEM

CLASSIFICATION	TYPICAL EXAMPLES	OTHER EXAMPLES
GENETIC DISORDERS Genetic disorders originate from a defect or defects in the inherited genetic material within a person's cells. In most cases, the defective genes are passed from the mother or father. But sometimes a genetic disorder occurs as a result of a new gene defect, because of the mutation of a gene. Genetic disorders may appear at birth or many years later.	Huntington's chorea is inherited in an autosomal dominant pattern, which means that it affects both sexes and manifests itself whenever a defective gene is inherited from either parent. Huntington's chorea does not usually appear until age 35 to 50. Characteristic features include uncontrollable, jerky movements (choreas), behavioral changes, and dementia. Symptoms result from a degeneration of the basal ganglia.	Fragile X syndrome Phenylketonuria Tay-Sachs disease Wilson's disease
DEVELOPMENTAL DISORDERS Developmental disorders originate from abnormal fetal development, not from defective genes. Known causes include viral infections or the use of alcohol, nicotine, or other drugs by the mother. Developmental disorders can sometimes be identified by ultrasound scanning during pregnancy.	In spina bifida, part of one or more of the vertebrae fails to develop, leaving a portion of the spinal cord exposed. In the most severe cases, the defect may cause paralysis of the legs and loss of bladder and bowel control. The cause of spina bifida is unknown.	Cerebral palsy (see page 129) Hydrocephalus (water on the brain) Anencephaly (absence of most of the brain) Microcephaly (small head)
IMPAIRED BLOOD AND OXYGEN SUPPLY The brain requires abundant oxygen and glucose and is exceptionally sensitive to any reduction in supply, even for a few minutes. Anything that interferes with the brain's blood supply or prevents oxygen from entering the blood can quickly cause brain damage.	During labor, a baby's umbilical cord can protrude through the mother's cervix, interfering with the baby's blood supply. In older people, the most frequent cause of impaired blood supply is cerebrovascular disease (see STROKE AND RELATED DISORDERS on page 106).	Heart attack Strangulation Asphyxiation Drowning Severe asthma attacks
PHYSICAL INJURY The brain and spinal cord are vulnerable to injury, especially if the skull or vertebral column is fractured. Injury may occur from the high-speed impact of a motor-vehicle accident, or from falls, sports injuries, bullet wounds, or other physical violence.	Skull fractures may cause direct damage to brain tissue. Bleeding from torn blood vessels into the spaces between the skull and brain may compress the brain. After brain injuries, scarring may cause seizures (see HEAD AND NECK INJURY on page 122).	Severed or cut nerves (see page 34) Spinal cord damage
INFECTION Almost any microorganism, including viruses, bacteria, fungi, and yeasts, can infect the brain, the membranes surrounding the brain and spinal cord (the meninges), or the spinal cord itself. Infection may enter the nervous system directly from a penetrating wound, may spread from a local infection, or may travel from another site by means of the bloodstream. Brain infection can develop into a brain abscess, which damages nerve tracts and impairs brain function.	Meningitis (inflammation of the meninges) may be caused by a virus or a bacterium. Viral meningitis, whose symptoms resemble those of influenza and include drowsiness and headache, is usually relatively mild. Bacterial meningitis is a serious illness that can be fatal in young children.	Rabies Poliomyelitis (polio) Syphilis (advanced stage) Acquired immunodeficiency syndrome (AIDS)
TUMORS Tumors can occur in any part of the brain or spinal cord or their coverings. In many cases, the tumors spread from sites elsewhere in the body. Tumors can directly destroy tissue or compress other structures as they grow within a limited space.	Brain tumors occur much more commonly than spinal cord tumors. Brain cancers usually spread, or metastasize, from cancers elsewhere in the body. Many types of benign (noncancerous) tumors may also seriously affect the brain (see BRAIN TUMORS on page 98).	

CLASSIFICATION	TYPICAL EXAMPLES	OTHER EXAMPLES
NEUROTRANSMITTER DISTURBANCE Numerous neurotransmitters (chemicals secreted by nerve cells to communicate with each other) exist in the brain and nervous system. Each serves a unique function. Brain and nervous system disorders can arise from altered production of a neurotransmitter, altered sensitivity of its specific receptor site (through which it affects other nerve cells), or selective loss of nerve cells that contain a particular neurotransmitter.	Certain types of severe depression seem to involve an underproduction in the brain of the neurotransmitters norepinephrine and serotonin. Depression can sometimes be treated with drugs that prevent the normal breakdown of either or both of these neurotransmitters (for example, phenelzine) or drugs that prolong their availability at the receptor site (for example, imipramine).	Parkinson's disease Alzheimer's disease Schizophrenia Huntington's chorea
DISORDERS OF THE BODY'S WHOLE SYSTEM The brain and nerves depend not only on a constant supply of oxygen and nutrients but also on closely controlled levels of acidity and constituents of the blood. Disorders of other body organs can lead to a breakdown of homeostasis (the mechanisms employed by the body to keep it in a steady, balanced state).	Severe diabetes mellitus, in which the pancreas fails to produce insulin, causes acid substances (ketone bodies) to accumulate in the body. Without regular insulin injections, these substances interfere with brain function, leading to coma and sometimes death.	Liver or kidney failure Disease or absence of the parathyroid glands
NERVE COMPRESSION FROM JOINT, SKELETAL, OR SOFT-TISSUE DISORDERS Compression or entrapment of a nerve or nerve root by surrounding structures can cause pain, numbness, or weakness in the area supplied by the nerve.	In carpal tunnel syndrome (see page 30), ligaments surrounding the wrist compress the median nerve. People with this disorder experience pain and numbness in the thumb and first two fingers. They also suffer weakness and shrinkage in portions of the hand.	Saturday night palsy (see page 30) Disc prolapse (slipped disc)
POISONING Many poisons can damage the brain and nervous system. Chronic poisoning occurs during long-term, gradual intake of small doses of a toxic substance (such as alcohol). Acute poisoning (such as food poisoning) happens when a large amount of poison enters or is produced in the body in a short time.	The gradual accumulation of environmental poisons, such as lead (see page 34), mercury, and arsenic, can also cause nervous system damage. Lead from leaded house paints is linked to mental retardation in children.	Drug abuse MPTP (a highly toxic by-product of illicit drugs; see page 117) Botulism Strychnine Toxins produced by diphtheria and tetanus
DEGENERATIVE DISORDERS Medical science has yet to discover the cause of these disorders. They are characterized by gradual, progressive degeneration of part of the nervous system. Many diseases previously thought to be degenerative, whose causes have since been identified, have been reclassified. Creutzfeldt-Jakob disease, which causes progressive dementia, is now known to result from a "slow-growing" virus – a viral infection that takes many years to develop.	A group of rare disorders called motor neuron disease causes weakness and wasting of muscles through degeneration of motor nerve cells in the brain and spinal cord. The most common type, amyotrophic lateral sclerosis (ALS, also known as Lou Gehrig's disease), usually affects people over age 50. Early signs include weakness in the hands and arms, which usually progresses to the muscles that control respiration and swallowing. Most people with ALS die within 2 to 4 years of diagnosis.	Parkinson's disease (see page 116) Multiple sclerosis (see page 130) Alzheimer's disease (see DEMENTIA on page 134) Huntington's chorea
DISORDERS OF UNKNOWN ORIGIN Some disorders are characterized by their symptoms or their effects on the brain rather than by any obvious cause. But effective treatment is available for some of these disorders, when doctors understand how their symptoms are produced.	Migraine produces recurrent, severe, throbbing pain over part of the head or its entirety. The release of certain chemicals – especially serotonin – from the brain and other tissues causes changes in blood flow to the vessels of the brain and scalp. These changes produce cyclical narrowing and widening of blood vessels, which causes the pain (see HEADACHE on page 100).	Epilepsy (see page 92)

SYMPTOMS OF BRAIN AND NERVOUS SYSTEM DISORDERS

Nervous system disorders can affect any part of the nervous system – brain, cranial nerves, spinal cord, or spinal nerves. The illustration below shows the wide variety of symptoms that can occur in brain and nervous system disorders. Of course, some of these symptoms often have other, less serious causes.

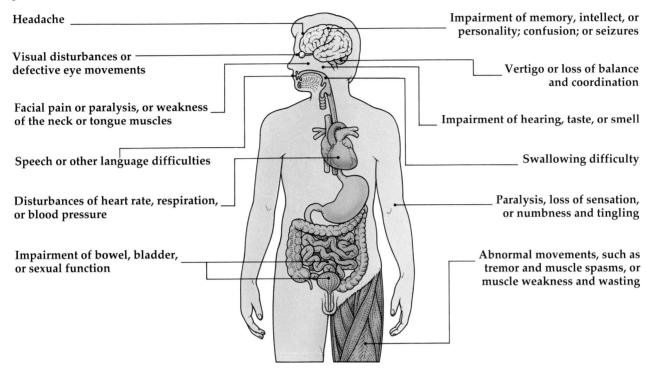

Headache

Visual disturbances or defective eye movements

Facial pain or paralysis, or weakness of the neck or tongue muscles

Speech or other language difficulties

Disturbances of heart rate, respiration, or blood pressure

Impairment of bowel, bladder, or sexual function

Impairment of memory, intellect, or personality; confusion; or seizures

Vertigo or loss of balance and coordination

Impairment of hearing, taste, or smell

Swallowing difficulty

Paralysis, loss of sensation, or numbness and tingling

Abnormal movements, such as tremor and muscle spasms, or muscle weakness and wasting

LEVELS OF CONSCIOUSNESS

In normal health, you experience a range of consciousness, from alertness, through drowsiness, to deep sleep. In various brain disorders, this continuum encompasses several abnormal levels, including brain death. The different stages of consciousness (normal and abnormal) and their key features are listed below.

Legal definition of brain death
To identify brain death, doctors first need to know that brain damage is irreversible. Then they check pupil, blink, gag, and respiratory reflexes. A lack of response indicates that the body's vital control centers in the brain stem no longer function. The vital bodily functions can be maintained only by artificial means. Brain death is the medical, legal, and ethical equivalent of death.

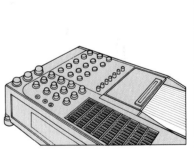

NORMAL STATES	ABNORMAL STATES		
1. Normal consciousness Awake; fully aware of self and environment; fully responsive to stimuli; level may fluctuate from full alertness to slight drowsiness.	**3. Confusion** Drowsy; clouded consciousness; disordered thought processes; short attention span; disorientation; poor memory; loss of bladder and bowel control; can be fully aroused; may be delirious.	**5. Light coma** Some response (grunting, coughing, or blinking) to vigorous stimulation; no spontaneous movements; spontaneous breathing.	**7. Vegetative state** May follow deep coma; eyes may be open; no awareness of surroundings; random purposeless movements; spontaneous breathing; no speech; no meaningful response to external stimuli.
2. Asleep Eyes closed; little or no awareness of self and surroundings; cessation of swallowing; responsive to external stimuli, such as shouting, pinching, or bright light; easily awakened.	**4. Stupor** Mental and physical activity is minimal; poor or absent response to spoken commands; aroused only by repeated, vigorous external stimuli; some spontaneous movements.	**6. Deep coma** No response to any external stimuli; no spontaneous movements; no speech; spontaneous breathing; eyes remain closed.	**8. Brain death** Irreversible state of deep coma; no spontaneous breathing; no spontaneous movement; no response to any stimulation; pupils unreactive; no electrical activity in brain.

INVESTIGATING NERVOUS SYSTEM DISORDERS

You probably don't realize it, but your doctor begins to examine your nervous system as soon as you walk into his or her office. Your doctor notices your speech, posture, handshake, balance, and gait, all of which provide clues about the state of your nervous system. He or she questions you to find out whether you or anyone in your family has had any previous nervous system problems. Then your doctor conducts a complete physical examination. If necessary, he or she will order further tests.

Mental status
First your doctor makes certain you are aware of the correct time and place. You may be asked to repeat certain phrases, name objects, or remember a series of words. You may also have to perform calculations, copy a drawn figure, or interpret proverbs.

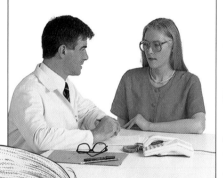

EXAMINING YOUR NERVOUS SYSTEM

The examination includes an evaluation of your mental status, cranial nerves, motor system, sensory system, and reflexes, as outlined below.

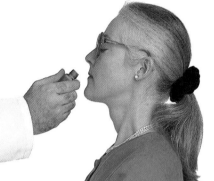

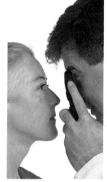

The 2nd cranial nerve
Your doctor examines the interior of your eyes with an instrument called an ophthalmoscope. He or she also tests various aspects of your vision, including visual fields.

The 1st cranial nerve
To check your sense of smell, your doctor tests whether you can identify different odors with your eyes closed.

The 3rd, 4th, and 6th cranial nerves
Your doctor inspects your eyelids, examines your eye movements, and shines a light into your pupils to test their contraction.

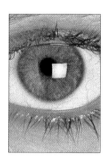

The 7th cranial nerve
Your doctor tests your facial movements. In some cases, he or she tests your sense of taste by applying certain substances to your tongue.

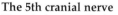

The 5th cranial nerve
Your doctor tests the function of your jaw muscles and your facial sensation. He or she tests the sensitivity of your corneas (the transparent coverings of your eyes) by touching them with a wisp of cotton.

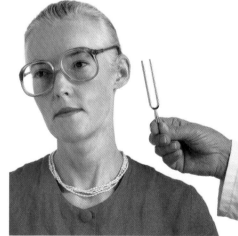

The 8th cranial nerve
Your doctor tests your ability to hear certain sounds and evaluates your ability to balance.

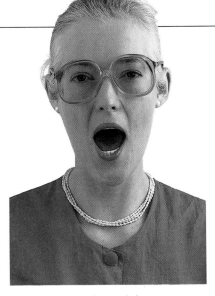

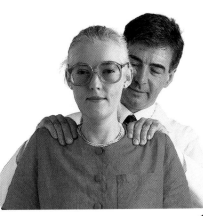

The 11th cranial nerve
Your doctor inspects the muscles in your neck and shoulders. He or she asks you to turn your head to each side against resistance and to shrug your shoulders against resistance.

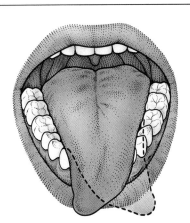

The 12th cranial nerve
Your doctor tests your tongue and its movements by asking you to stick out your tongue and to move it from side to side freely and against resistance.

The 9th and 10th cranial nerves
Your doctor checks your speech and inspects your palate to determine whether its movements are normal.

Examining your sensory system
While your eyes are closed, your doctor tests your touch, pain, temperature, position, and vibration sensations. Such tests include brushing your skin lightly with cotton and pricking it gently with a sterile pin. Your doctor may also test your ability to identify certain objects by their shapes.

Examining your motor system
Your doctor examines your muscles to identify abnormal movements and checks muscle tone. He or she tests the muscle power in your arms and legs. You will grip your doctor's hands and move your limbs against resistance. Your doctor also tests your coordination. He or she watches you walk and may ask you to walk on your toes or heel to toe.

Testing reflexes
Your doctor tests your knee, ankle, biceps (front upper arm muscle), and triceps (back upper arm muscle) reflexes by tapping the tendons with a small hammer. He or she draws a pointed object up the side of your foot and observes how your toes move in response. Several other reflexes are usually examined as well.

FURTHER INVESTIGATION

If your doctor finds possible evidence of a nervous system disorder, he or she may refer you for more tests to help diagnose the problem. These tests may include:

◆Electroencephalography (EEG): recordings of electrical activity in the brain

◆Evoked potentials: measurements of the brain's electrical activity in response to auditory, sensory, or visual stimuli

◆Nerve conduction studies: electrical stimulation of a nerve to test its function

◆Biopsy: removal and analysis of tissue

◆Biochemical tests and blood cell counts: tests of blood serum (component of blood) and blood cells

◆ CT scan (see page 90): an imaging test to look at the brain or spinal cord

◆ MRI (see page 90): an imaging test of the brain or spinal cord that is more sensitive than CT scanning for some abnormalities

◆Lumbar puncture: removal of a small amount of spinal fluid

◆Audiometry: tests of the sense of hearing

◆Electromyography: recordings of the electrical activity of a muscle to detect nerve or muscle disorders

DIAGNOSING PROBLEMS: IMAGING THE LIVING BRAIN

Some techniques enable doctors to actually see inside the living brain. These technologies help doctors diagnose brain disorders more accurately than ever before. X-rays enable limited investigation of brain structure. Doctors can learn more through techniques such as ventriculography, in which air is introduced into the brain ventricles (cavities), and angiography, in which an opaque dye is injected into the brain's circulation. But both of these methods present risks for the patient. In recent years, these techniques have been largely replaced by more sophisticated imaging techniques: computed tomography (CT) scanning, magnetic resonance imaging (MRI), and positron emission tomography (PET).

How does CT scanning work?

CT scanning produces detailed X-ray images of the brain. A series of narrow, concentrated X-ray beams is passed through the head toward a type of photographic material that is more sensitive than X-ray film. Computer analysis of the exposed material enables the technician to create a cross-sectional image – much like a "slice" – that shows segments of skull bone and the brain's gray and white matter, blood vessels, cerebrospinal fluid, and any obvious neurological disorders.

How does PET scanning work?

PET scanning produces images of radioactive compounds (radionuclides) that reach brain tissues after injection or inhalation. The scanner detects radiation emitted, and a computer then constructs an image of the brain. Doctors use PET scanning to investigate the brain structures involved in nervous system disorders. This technique can show abnormal tissue, such as a tumor, and differentiate it from other abnormalities, such as scar tissue from surgery.

How does MRI work?

MRI produces high-quality images of organs and structures inside the body without X-rays or other radiation. Certain atomic particles emit specific radiofrequency signals when displaced by radio waves in a special magnetic field. By focusing on these signals, an MRI scan creates brain images showing much greater detail than those produced by either PET or CT scanning. MRI is now the imaging technique most doctors use to diagnose disorders such as brain cancer and multiple sclerosis.

How does angiography work?

Dye through which X-rays cannot pass is injected into a blood vessel that carries blood to the brain. The high degree of contrast caused by the dye on the resulting X-ray allows doctors to view detailed images of the blood vessels in the brain. Doctors use this technique to investigate cerebrovascular disease and tumor. Angiography is performed before surgery on the blood vessels. Because it can be dangerous, doctors use it with caution.

CT scan

In this CT scan, a brain tumor (arrow) is shown in the back of the right cerebral hemisphere. Left untreated, a brain tumor can lead to brain damage and even death.

PET scan

The color-enhanced PET scan below shows the lack of brain activity (black areas) in the left hemisphere after a massive stroke. The most active brain areas appear red and yellow.

MRI scan

This color-enhanced MRI scan reveals a cerebral infarct – an area of dead brain tissue caused by obstruction of crucial blood flow – in the right hemisphere (arrow).

Angiogram

This color-enhanced angiogram reveals an aneurysm (swelling) in an artery inside the skull (arrow). The swelling could rupture, but it can be corrected by surgery.

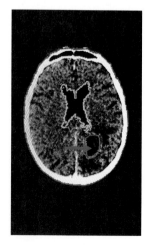
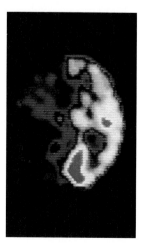
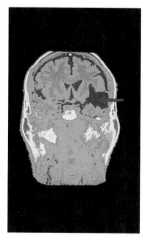
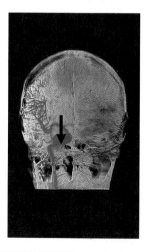

CASE HISTORY
SPREADING NUMBNESS

J ILL HAS ALWAYS **taken pride in her good health and excellent physical fitness. One day, while teaching a dance class, Jill experienced a pain in her lower back. This pain was so unusual that she stopped moving and stood still for some time, to the surprise of her pupils. The pain worsened and she had to leave the class. She made an appointment to see her doctor the same day.**

PERSONAL DETAILS
Name Jill Pozner
Age 27
Occupation Dance teacher
Family Both parents are healthy.

THE CONSULTATION
The doctor examines Jill but does not find anything wrong. He tells her that she has probably developed back strain from overexertion and recommends a day or two in bed.

Jill reluctantly complies. The next morning, she notices that both her feet are numb and tingling. She gets out of bed and starts her usual morning stretching routine. To her distress, she finds she cannot stand on her toes and seems to have no strength in her calf muscles. She goes back to bed. By evening, her buttocks and the fronts of both thighs have also become numb. The next morning, when she tries to stand, her legs give way and she collapses. She pulls herself onto her bed and calls her doctor. Within an hour, Jill is in the emergency room.

FURTHER INVESTIGATION
Jill's doctor orders a lumbar puncture to obtain a sample of cerebrospinal fluid from her spine. Analysis of the fluid shows no blood or other obvious abnormality. But an MRI scan of her spine reveals a slight swelling of the spinal cord at the level of the middle of her back.

THE DIAGNOSIS
By evening, both Jill's legs are paralyzed. The next day, she has no sensation in either leg or in the lower part of her trunk and has lost bladder control. The doctors conclude that Jill has suffered a severe inflammatory disorder affecting a limited area of her spinal cord. They make a diagnosis of ACUTE TRANSVERSE MYELITIS. The condition often occurs without obvious causes. The doctors tell Jill that as the acute stage passes, she may expect some recovery but that this cannot be guaranteed.

THE TREATMENT
The doctor prescribes large doses of a corticosteroid drug – an anti-inflammatory agent. After 3 weeks, Jill's symptoms begin to subside, and the drug treatment is stopped. The doctor tells Jill that people sometimes have a relapse at this stage, but Jill continues to make a slow recovery.

THE FOLLOW-UP
Jill continues to regain feeling and strength. After 6 months, Jill can walk and run and has recovered bladder control. But her legs remain weak. The doctors tell Jill to anticipate further strengthening of her muscles with regular use. She begins a fitness regimen and practices her dancing exercises daily.

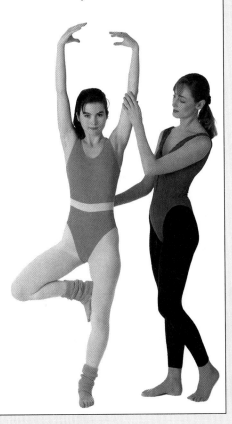

A new interest
Jill cannot dance with as much coordination as before. But she is able to continue teaching and begins to develop a greater interest in choreography.

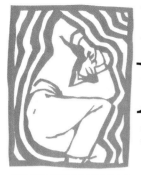

EPILEPSY

E PILEPSY is one of the most common serious neurological disorders. In many cases, epilepsy has no apparent cause but can result from such factors as head injury, a tumor, or a developmental abnormality. Currently, about 1 million people in the US are diagnosed as having epilepsy.

WHAT CAUSES EPILEPSY?

In many people, especially those with generalized seizures, doctors can find no clear cause of epilepsy. Strokes, head injury, tumors, or alcohol abuse are common causes when seizures develop in adults. In children, genetic diseases, developmental abnormalities, infections, and tumors head the list of possible causes of epileptic seizure.

A person with epilepsy tends to have some form of recurrent seizure, a sudden episode of unregulated electrical activity in the brain. The incidence of epilepsy varies considerably with age. Rates are highest in early childhood, lowest in early adult life, and increased in the elderly. Males are slightly more at risk. Some people with epilepsy have only a few seizures in a lifetime. Others may experience many seizures a day. Isolated seizures are common. In fact, about one person in 20 has a seizure some time during his or her life.

WHAT IS EPILEPSY?

All forms of epilepsy arise from a temporary malfunction, usually in one area of the brain. During an epileptic seizure, the brain's orderly flow of electrical signals is disturbed by abnormal electrical discharges. The type of epileptic seizure that occurs depends on the area affected and the pattern in which it spreads. Although there are many types of seizures, they can be divided into two broad categories: generalized and partial seizures.

Brain activity during a generalized seizure
Generalized seizures happen when electrical disturbances in a deep brain structure spread to the entire brain. This abnormal brain activity affects the whole body and results in loss of consciousness. Electroencephalograms (EEGs) recorded during a generalized seizure often show abnormal patterns like the one below, obtained during a grand mal seizure.

Normal EEG

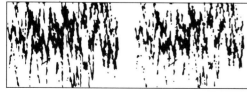

EEG recorded during grand mal seizure

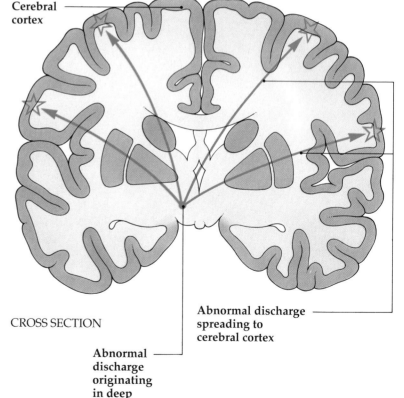

Cerebral cortex

CROSS SECTION

Abnormal discharge originating in deep brain structure

Abnormal discharge spreading to cerebral cortex

Disturbance remaining localized

Cerebral cortex

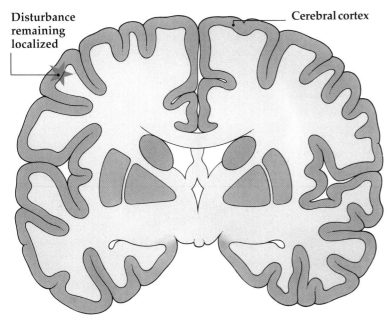

CROSS SECTION

Brain activity during a partial seizure
Electrical disturbances arise from a single location in the brain. The abnormal discharge remains localized and only affects isolated bodily or mental functions. Consciousness is not lost. Temporal lobe epilepsy is the best known type of simple partial seizure. During complex partial seizures, effects are widespread and often impair consciousness. If the effects spread widely enough, a generalized seizure may occur similar to a grand mal seizure. EEG tracings recorded during partial seizures often show spindlelike abnormalities, as shown below.

Normal EEG

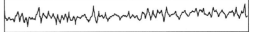

EEG recorded during a simple partial seizure

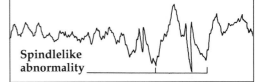

Spindlelike abnormality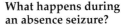

Generalized seizures

The two leading types of generalized seizures are grand mal, meaning "great sickness," and petit mal, or "little sickness." Today, petit mal seizures are more commonly called "absence seizures." The person experiences a momentary loss of consciousness without abnormal movements. This type of seizure occurs mainly in children (see caption at right).

Occasionally, people who have grand mal seizures experience a warning sensation, known as an "aura," which may be characterized by a hallucinatory sound or smell, abdominal discomfort, or a feeling of fullness in the head. In other cases, seizures occur without warning. At the outset of a grand mal seizure, the person loses consciousness and falls to the ground. The person's body stiffens, and breathing may be interrupted. Twitching or jerking may then begin, and the person may clench his or her teeth. As the shaking ceases, loss of bladder control may occur. After the seizure, the person may remain unconscious for up to 15 minutes. When consciousness returns, the person is confused and drowsy, and frequently has a

headache. He or she may then sleep for hours. Usually, the person remembers only the aura. If a succession of grand mal seizures occurs without recovery of consciousness, a condition known as status epilepticus, immediate medical attention is required. The person may die if the seizures do not stop.

What happens during an absence seizure?
Absence seizures, which mainly affect children, are so inconspicuous that they often pass unnoticed. For periods of a few seconds to up to half a minute, the affected person experiences a disruption in consciousness and becomes completely unaware. He or she may stare blankly ahead and stop talking. Small movements of the eyes or eyelids sometimes occur. Seizures may occur hundreds of times daily, affecting school performance. In rare cases, absence seizures are caused by tumors or identifiable brain diseases.

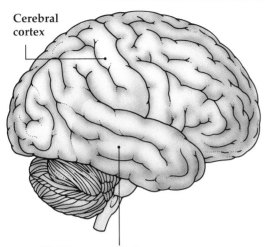

Cerebral cortex

Right temporal lobe

Temporal lobe epilepsy
The temporal lobes analyze sensory information and store memories. When the function of the right or left temporal lobe is disrupted in temporal lobe epilepsy (a type of partial seizure disorder), strange psychological phenomena may occur, including auditory, olfactory, or visual hallucinations and memory disturbance.

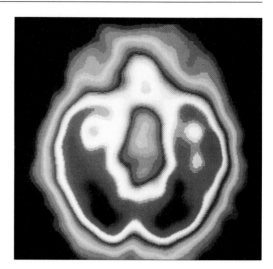

Partial seizures

Simple partial seizures occur without warning. Twitching movements may be accompanied by tingling sensations; numbness; an illusion of flashing lights; hallucinations of smell, hearing, and taste; nausea; and loss of balance. The person remains conscious throughout.

Complex partial seizures impair consciousness. These seizures generate hallucinations and sometimes a clear memory of preceding events. The person feels afraid and can become angry. He or she often behaves like a robot, repeatedly chewing, sucking, or swallowing. Attempts to restrain the person can cause a violent outburst.

DIAGNOSIS

Doctors can sometimes diagnose epilepsy simply by taking a medical history and performing a physical examination. Because the affected person may not recall what happened during a suspected seizure, doctors often question witnesses. Physical signs, such as injury to the body or tongue sustained during a seizure, strongly suggest grand mal epilepsy.

Prolonged EEG studies can show specific changes in brain activity, but their results do not always confirm a diagnosis of epilepsy. Some people with epilepsy have normal EEG patterns, and people without epilepsy occasionally

have abnormal patterns. A doctor may request MRI or CT scanning to rule out a tumor or other abnormalities.

TREATMENT

Epilepsy with an obvious underlying cause may cease once the cause has been treated. In about 75 percent of cases, seizures can be completely controlled or their frequency reduced with anticonvulsant drugs. Commonly used drugs include phenytoin, phenobarbital, carbamazepine, and valproic acid.

Positron emission tomography (PET) scanning
Doctors obtain PET scans (example shown above) to study brain function in people with epilepsy. Computed tomography (CT) scanning or magnetic resonance imaging (MRI) helps to locate structural damage.

Ambulatory EEG monitors
Doctors sometimes use an ambulatory EEG monitor, shown here, to investigate the possibility of epilepsy in people with fairly frequent seizures. This device increases the chance of recording brain impulses during an actual seizure. Electrocardiographic (ECG) studies of heart rhythms may also be performed in the elderly to find out whether cardiac irregularities are causing loss of consciousness or seizures.

CASE HISTORY
SEIZURES AND BEHAVIOR PROBLEMS

W HEN FRANKLIN was 2 years old, he was in a traffic accident that caused a concussion and bruising of his head. Doctors found no evidence of brain damage or skull fracture at the time. A few years later, Franklin suffered a series of grand mal seizures without recovering consciousness between seizures – a condition known as status epilepticus. Franklin's parents called an ambulance and he was rushed to the hospital.

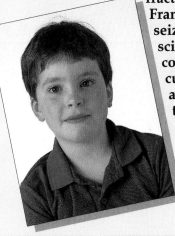

PERSONAL DETAILS
Name Franklin Bertorini
Age 6
Occupation Student
Family No history of significant disease.

MEDICAL BACKGROUND
Franklin had a normal birth and, until the traffic accident occurred, had not experienced any serious injuries or illnesses.

EMERGENCY TREATMENT
The emergency room team immediately gives Franklin an injection of the sedative drug diazepam to stop his seizures, followed by the anticonvulsant drug phenytoin for longer-term control.

THE INVESTIGATIONS
At the hospital, an examination of Franklin's nervous system reveals no definite abnormality. An EEG tracing shows a number of low points on the left side of his brain that are emitting large electrical spikes, but a CT scan is normal. The neurologist explains that Franklin has developed a seizure disorder and prescribes daily doses of phenytoin. He asks Franklin's parents to bring him in for regular checkups.

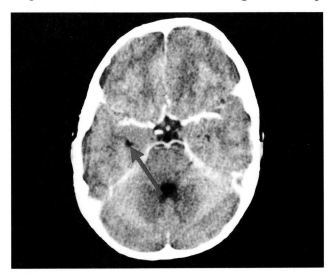

Identifying the problem
A CT scan of Franklin's brain, shown here, reveals an area of scarring (arrow) in the left temporal lobe, possibly caused by the head injury he received in a traffic accident.

Later, Franklin's parents report that he continues to have partial seizures during which he complains of a bad smell and experiences visual hallucinations. During a typical seizure, he repeatedly turns his head and eyes to the right and makes chewing and swallowing movements. This automatic behavior is occasionally followed by a grand mal seizure, but more frequently Franklin simply seems to be unaware of his surroundings. When Franklin's parents attempt to interrupt or control his behavior, he cries or runs away.

THE DIAGNOSIS
The neurologist tells Franklin's parents that the behavior they describe is a seizure, typical of TEMPORAL LOBE EPILEPSY, which sometimes becomes more widespread, resulting in a grand mal seizure. Over the course of a few years, the doctor prescribes different anticonvulsant drugs, but Franklin's seizures continue.

FURTHER INVESTIGATION AND TREATMENT
The doctor decides to refer Franklin for another CT scan, which reveals, for the first time, an area of scarring (sclerosis) in the left temporal area of his brain. This scarring could have originated from the injury Franklin received in the traffic accident. Franklin undergoes more detailed EEG testing, during which electrodes are surgically inserted into his brain by a neurosurgeon. Franklin then has brain surgery to remove the damaged area that is probably causing the seizures.

THE OUTCOME
To his parents' relief, Franklin's seizures stop and his behavior improves dramatically after surgery. His teachers report that he is progressing well in school.

Doctors must carefully adjust dosage in anticonvulsant therapy. Sometimes combination drug therapy yields better results than single-drug therapy. After a person has been seizure-free for at least 2 years, doctors can often withdraw medication, occasionally with no recurrence of seizures. Withdrawal of anticonvulsants should never be attempted without medical advice.

Surgery may improve epilepsy, but removal of a brain tumor or an abscess does not always completely eliminate seizures that originate from such disorders. About one third of patients who have simple or complex partial seizures stop experiencing epileptic seizures once specific areas of damage in the brain have been surgically removed (see CASE HISTORY on page 95).

LIVING WITH EPILEPSY

Complying with medical treatment is the best way people with epilepsy can control the disorder. But people who have epilepsy can take additional steps to successfully manage their condition.

Identifying trigger factors

Life-style factors sometimes prompt seizures. Many epileptics find that lack of sleep, a high fever, excess alcohol intake, or emotional disturbances provoke seizures. People with epilepsy should get plenty of sleep and try to avoid stress as much as possible.

Some people have a rare form of epilepsy triggered by exposure to specific physical stimuli, such as a flickering

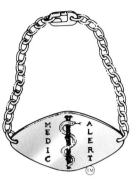

Alerting others to the condition
A person with epilepsy may choose to wear a special bracelet or carry a card or tag to alert others to his or her condition in the event of a seizure. An epileptic should tell colleagues and friends what steps to take if a seizure occurs in their presence.

FIRST AID FOR AN EPILEPTIC SEIZURE

Witnessing a major (grand mal) seizure can be distressing, but it is important not to overreact. Seizures generally last only a minute or two and are not life-threatening unless they occur in a dangerous place. If you should ever be present during a seizure, let it run its course. Make sure that the person is in no danger of falling or being hurt by furniture and that he or she can breathe while unconscious.

4 Once jerking movements have stopped, wait for the person to regain consciousness and then find a quiet place for him or her to rest. It is normal for the person to feel dazed and confused for an hour or more after the seizure.

What to do :

1 If there is warning that a seizure is about to occur, or if the person is about to fall, help the person lie down in a safe place.

2 If he or she has already fallen, remove objects or furniture from the area to prevent physical injury. Do not attempt to move the person unless he or she has fallen in a dangerous place.

3 Loosen tight clothing around the person's neck and place soft padding under his or her head. Do not attempt to restrain the person's movements and do not place anything in his or her mouth or try to open it. If the person vomits, try to turn his or her head to allow drainage.

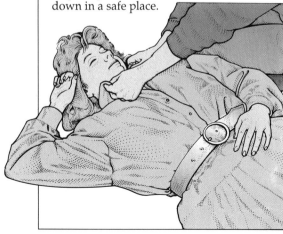

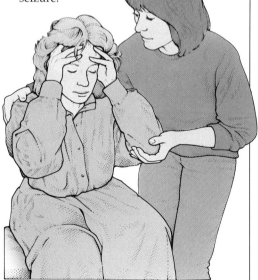

5 If the seizure continues for more than 5 minutes, if a second seizure immediately follows the first, or if serious physical injury may have occurred, call an ambulance.

Exercise and epilepsy
People with epilepsy can and should exercise regularly. But people whose seizures are not completely controlled should avoid obviously dangerous activities, such as rock climbing or swimming alone. Sports with a high risk of head injury, such as boxing, should also be avoided.

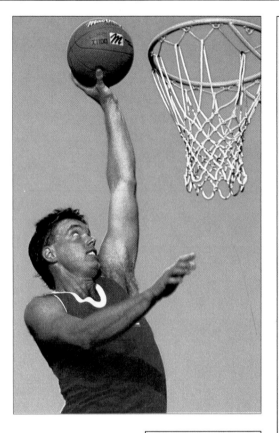

light or certain types of music. A person with this form of epilepsy can learn to use a distraction technique, which diverts attention from the stimulus, as a way of preventing such seizures.

Coping psychologically

A person with epilepsy may need some time to accept any limitations imposed by the disorder. The person often finds it easier to cope with the management of seizures than with other people's attitudes about the condition. The support of family, friends, and colleagues is extremely important. Overprotection of a child with epilepsy is common but it can adversely affect the way the child matures and socializes.

Feelings of inferiority or self-consciousness may arise as a result of seizures. Epilepsy support groups offer advice and support and can bolster confidence. Some people find psychotherapy more personal and helpful. Vocational centers help epileptics secure training and find employment.

DRIVING AND WORKING RESTRICTIONS

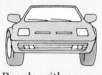

People with a seizure disorder such as epilepsy are not issued a driver's license in the US unless their seizures have been kept under control for at least two years. People whose epilepsy is incompletely controlled should not operate unguarded machinery or work at heights. Employability may be reduced by these restrictions. The best way to control seizures is to comply with medical treatment.

ASK YOUR DOCTOR
EPILEPSY

Q **My son has been diagnosed as having epilepsy. Can he have a seizure in his sleep?**

A Yes, but having an epileptic seizure during sleep is no more dangerous than experiencing one while awake. Your son may not even be aware that the seizure has occurred. There is a possibility that he might not be near anyone should he need help, but his chances of being injured from a fall are greatly reduced.

Q **Is there any reason to fear that my husband's epilepsy will shorten his life span?**

A Unless your husband's epilepsy is caused by a serious underlying condition, such as a brain tumor or advanced kidney disease, it should not shorten his life span. It is important, however, for him to receive appropriate medical treatment. If his doctor thinks it is necessary, your husband should avoid situations such as driving or engaging in certain sports.

Q **If I become pregnant, could the anticonvulsant drugs I have been taking harm my baby?**

A Several studies have shown a slight but definite increase in the incidence of birth defects in babies born to women receiving anticonvulsant therapy. No anticonvulsant drugs are considered entirely safe, but the risks of seizures in pregnant women with uncontrolled epilepsy far outweigh the risk of an abnormality in the baby caused by the drug. Ask a neurologist to discuss potential risks with you before you attempt to conceive.

BRAIN TUMORS

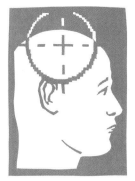

NOT ALL BRAIN tumors are malignant (cancerous), but they are always serious. A tumor may interfere with the normal circulation of the cerebrospinal fluid, and areas of the brain adjoining the tumor can become compressed or destroyed as the tumor grows. Because the skull is made of bone, the growing tumor cannot expand, causing pressure to build.

TYPES OF TUMORS

Primary brain tumors arise from tissues inside the skull. They include:

◆ **Gliomas** from the supporting cells of the brain
◆ **Meningiomas** from the membranes that cover the brain
◆ **Pituitary tumors**
◆ **Acoustic neuromas**

Secondary tumors arise from tumors in other parts of the body.

The dangerous rise in pressure caused by a brain tumor produces some common symptoms: severe, persistent headaches; sudden and unexpected vomiting; visual disturbances, such as loss of part of the field of vision; and hallucinations, personality changes, or sudden onset of abnormal and uncharacteristic behavior. Compression of brain tissue can trigger epileptic seizures, which may be generalized or confined to involuntary movements of one side of the body.

DIAGNOSIS AND TREATMENT

A doctor may notice one sign of a brain tumor during an examination of the eyes with an instrument called an ophthal-moscope. Swelling or protrusion of the optic discs (the parts of the optic nerves visible within the eyes) provides evidence of increased pressure in the skull, possibly because of a tumor in the brain. The doctor can usually confirm the diagnosis by computed tomography (CT) scanning or magnetic resonance imaging (MRI). These techniques can also determine the exact site of the tumor and can establish its size and extent of spread.

Many common brain tumors are not malignant. Cure comes with complete surgical removal of the tumor. If surgeons cannot completely remove a tumor, they cut away as much of it as possible. Doctors may supplement surgery for a malignant tumor with radiation therapy or anticancer drugs.

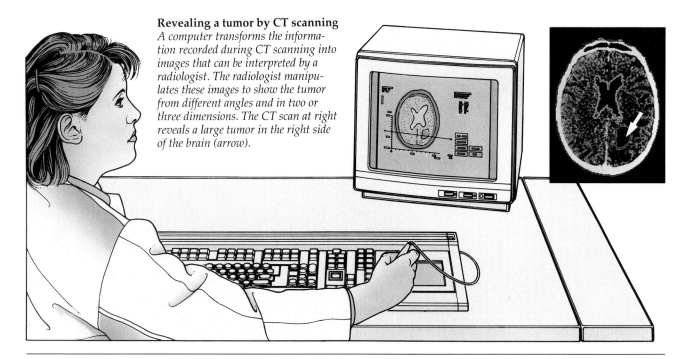

Revealing a tumor by CT scanning
A computer transforms the information recorded during CT scanning into images that can be interpreted by a radiologist. The radiologist manipulates these images to show the tumor from different angles and in two or three dimensions. The CT scan at right reveals a large tumor in the right side of the brain (arrow).

SURGICAL PROCEDURES
STEREOTAXIC SURGERY

ODAY, **many operations to investigate and treat brain tumors are performed with delicate instruments inserted through a tiny, surgically created hole in the skull. Imaging techniques such as CT scanning or MRI enable the surgeon to locate diseased brain structures and to guide instruments precisely to a targeted area. Surgeons may use stereotaxic surgery to obtain a biopsy specimen (small sample of tissue) or to remove the tumor. The procedure also permits tumor treatment through the implantation of radioactive seeds (tiny pellets of a radioactive substance) or laser or ultrasound destruction of the tumor.**

1 During general or local anesthesia, the surgeon attaches an adjustable metal frame to the patient's skull.

2 The surgical team obtains CT scans to identify the precise area to be treated. A computer calculates the best position for the insertion of instruments. A three-dimensional image, as shown here, is sometimes used to help the surgeon determine the tumor's volume and location.

Tumor

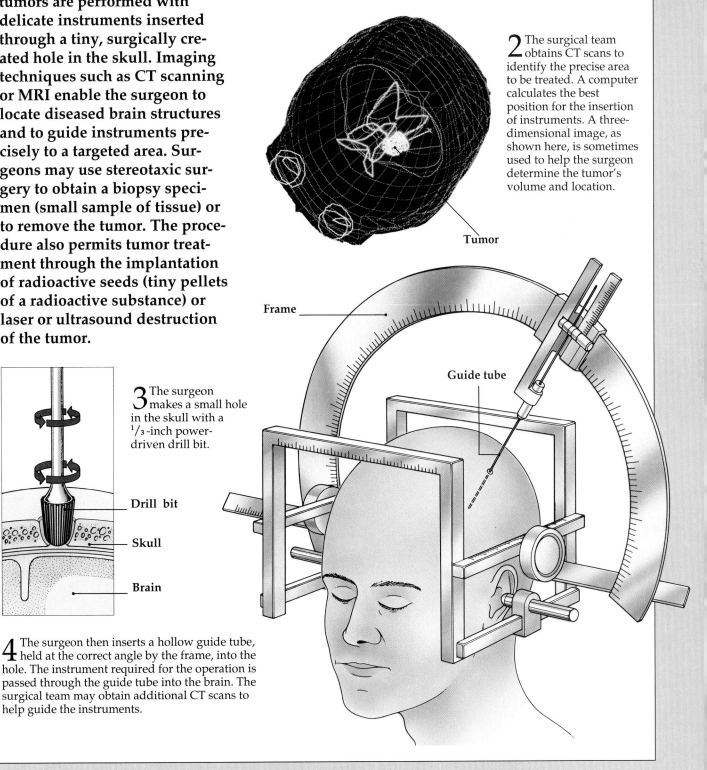

Frame

Guide tube

3 The surgeon makes a small hole in the skull with a $^{1}/_{3}$-inch power-driven drill bit.

Drill bit

Skull

Brain

4 The surgeon then inserts a hollow guide tube, held at the correct angle by the frame, into the hole. The instrument required for the operation is passed through the guide tube into the brain. The surgical team may obtain additional CT scans to help guide the instruments.

HEADACHES

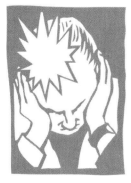

T HEY PIERCE, pound, and throb. They make you feel like your head is in a vise, or like a jackhammer is pulsating inside your skull. They're headaches, and they strike more than 90 percent of the US population. Most people have headaches only occasionally. But millions suffer recurrent headaches. Despite their frequency, we have yet to find a universally effective way to ease the pain.

Many factors can bring on an occasional, ordinary headache. (Some of the most common causes are listed at left.) Recurrent headaches often arise from migraine or from muscle tension in the scalp, neck, or face. Recurrent headaches develop gradually, clear up in a few hours to a day, and have no serious aftereffects. Tension headaches may become chronic (constant or long term).

Doctors designate some recurrent headaches as specific diseases – including migraine and its variants: cluster headache and paroxysmal hemicrania (severe, one-sided headache). Although migraine sufferers have a painful and sometimes incapacitating disorder, they usually tolerate their discomfort without needing hospitalization. While the variants of migraine mentioned above are not dangerous, relief of symptoms sometimes requires intensive treatment or even hospitalization.

MIGRAINE

The word migraine comes from the Greek word "hemicrania," meaning "half the head." The severe, recurring pain of migraine is aggravated by light and is often accompanied by nausea and vomiting. Migraine affects 5 to 10 percent of the population and occurs more commonly in women. Often inherited, migraine usually starts during the teenage years or in early adult life. Recurrent, severe headaches that begin in middle age or later may be due to another cause.

ORDINARY HEADACHES

Common, ordinary headaches can be brought on by:

◆ Muscle strain or injury
◆ Stress
◆ Too little or too much sleep
◆ Overeating
◆ Excessive alcohol consumption
◆ A noisy or a poorly ventilated environment
◆ Prolonged concentration
◆ Eye strain
◆ Jaw tension
◆ Poor posture

What to do:

Take a painkiller, such as acetaminophen or aspirin (do not give aspirin to children or adolescents). Relax with your eyes closed.

Infection
A headache may originate from increased pressure inside the skull due to the swelling produced by a brain infection (encephalitis) or from infection and inflammation of the membranes that surround the brain and spinal cord (meningitis).

Meninges (membranes that surround the brain and spinal cord)

Temporal arteritis
Inflammation of the main scalp artery (the temporal artery) may occur in the elderly, causing pain in one temple. Untreated, this disorder can affect other arteries, sometimes leading to partial or total blindness.

Muscles of the scalp

Temporal artery

Temple

Muscles of the neck

Chronic tension headache
This type of long-lasting or recurring headache originates partly from muscular tension in the head and neck.

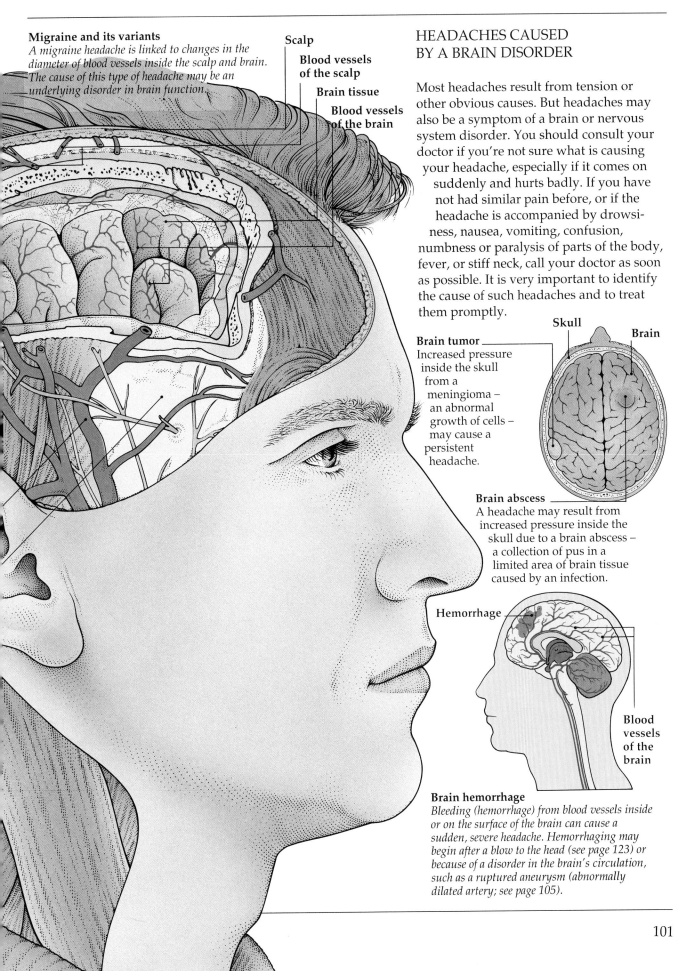

Migraine and its variants
A migraine headache is linked to changes in the diameter of blood vessels inside the scalp and brain. The cause of this type of headache may be an underlying disorder in brain function.

Scalp

Blood vessels of the scalp

Brain tissue

Blood vessels of the brain

HEADACHES CAUSED BY A BRAIN DISORDER

Most headaches result from tension or other obvious causes. But headaches may also be a symptom of a brain or nervous system disorder. You should consult your doctor if you're not sure what is causing your headache, especially if it comes on suddenly and hurts badly. If you have not had similar pain before, or if the headache is accompanied by drowsiness, nausea, vomiting, confusion, numbness or paralysis of parts of the body, fever, or stiff neck, call your doctor as soon as possible. It is very important to identify the cause of such headaches and to treat them promptly.

Skull

Brain

Brain tumor
Increased pressure inside the skull from a meningioma – an abnormal growth of cells – may cause a persistent headache.

Brain abscess
A headache may result from increased pressure inside the skull due to a brain abscess – a collection of pus in a limited area of brain tissue caused by an infection.

Hemorrhage

Blood vessels of the brain

Brain hemorrhage
Bleeding (hemorrhage) from blood vessels inside or on the surface of the brain can cause a sudden, severe headache. Hemorrhaging may begin after a blow to the head (see page 123) or because of a disorder in the brain's circulation, such as a ruptured aneurysm (abnormally dilated artery; see page 105).

101

HEADACHES CAUSED BY OTHER UNDERLYING DISORDERS

Many health problems other than brain or nervous system disorders can bring on headache pain. Consult your doctor if you suspect your headaches might be caused by any of these common problems.

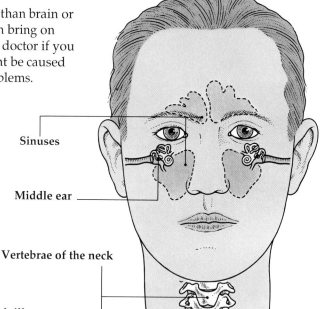

Ear problems
Infection of the middle ear (otitis media) can cause a headache.

Cervical osteoarthritis
In this condition, which is particularly common in the elderly, the joints that link the vertebrae in the neck compress the cervical (neck) nerves. This constriction causes pain in the neck region that spreads up the back of the scalp.

Sinuses

Middle ear

Vertebrae of the neck

Feverish illness
Headache is a common symptom of a cold or influenza (flu).

Glaucoma
Glaucoma – increased pressure within the eye – can cause a headache along with blurred vision and inflammation of the eye. Glaucoma is rare before the age of 40. Left untreated, it can lead to impairment of vision.

Visual disorders
Headaches occasionally arise from vision problems, such as deterioration of focusing ability, clouding of the eye lens (cataract), or an eye disease.

Sinusitis
Inflammation of the membrane that lines the sinuses – the cavities in the facial bones – may cause a headache, usually felt as facial pain. After a cold, infection can spread from the nose into the sinuses, causing inflammation and pain.

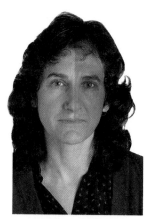

Common migraine
Common migraine is characterized by severe pain affecting half of the head or the entire head. Warning symptoms precede each attack. Migraine lasts for hours but can continue as long as a few days. The pain is usually throbbing and often produces scalp tenderness.

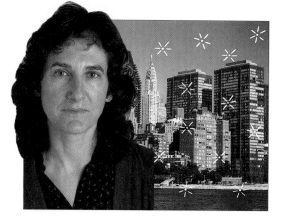

Classic migraine
Classic migraine headache symptoms duplicate those of common migraine. But just before onset, the person experiences a neurological symptom, such as a visual disturbance: flashing or sparkling lights, colored patterns, distortion or fragmentation of visual images, and small areas of blindness.

Types of migraine

Migraine attacks take different forms in different people. Attacks of migraine are often grouped into three categories: common migraine and classic migraine, which account for the majority of attacks, and complicated migraine. The characteristics of common and classic migraine are described at left. Complicated migraine attacks leave the person with a disturbance of brain function, which produces such symptoms as tingling or weakness on one side of the body, loss of speech, or double vision due to disturbed eye movements. These disturbances, which arise in areas of the brain supplied by branches of the internal carotid arteries, may persist for a short time after the migraine headache is gone. One rare form of complicated migraine brings on headache with dizziness, ringing in the ears, confusion, and, occasionally, loss of consciousness. This type of migraine affects the basilar artery, which supplies blood to the base of the brain.

Treating migraine

If you have severe headaches and experience accompanying symptoms, such as limb weakness, your doctor will want to make certain you do not have a more serious disorder. Once migraine has been accurately diagnosed, the first step in its treatment is to identify and eliminate factors that are likely to precipitate an attack. Trigger factors, the most common of which are listed at right, vary among migraine sufferers. If you have migraine headaches, you might find it useful to keep a headache diary to find out whether a certain action, such as eliminating cheese, chocolate, or red wine from your diet or discontinuing the oral contraceptive pill, affects the frequency of migraine attacks.

Painkillers such as acetaminophen or aspirin sometimes relieve symptoms. It is important that the painkiller be taken at the earliest sign of an attack. Anti-nausea drugs such as prochlorperazine can be taken to relieve nausea and vomiting. When simple painkillers do not work, ergotamine, which constricts the dilated blood vessels surrounding and within the brain, often provides relief. This drug is available in tablet, suppository, inhaler, and injectable forms. Migraine sufferers should keep a small supply of the preferred drug to use at the onset of warning symptoms. Most people find that they can recover more quickly if they can go to sleep in a darkened room.

Some migraine attacks are so frequent and the pain so severe that hospitalization is required. Doctors usually must keep the hospitalized person sedated, and intravenous replacement of fluids lost through vomiting becomes necessary. The person usually recovers in a few days.

Drugs such as amitriptyline, propranolol, or methysergide are used to prevent frequent attacks of migraine. Some people have also used relaxation and biofeedback techniques to find relief.

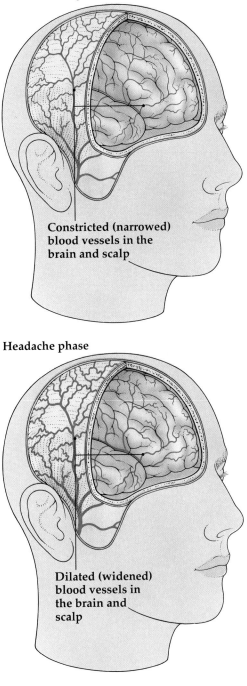

Onset of a migraine attack

Constricted (narrowed) blood vessels in the brain and scalp

Headache phase

Dilated (widened) blood vessels in the brain and scalp

What happens during migraine?
Abnormal changes in the diameter of blood vessels in both the scalp and the brain seem to produce the symptoms of migraine. These blood vessels narrow at the onset of an attack when visual or other neurological disturbances of classic migraine occur. Other vessels in the scalp and brain widen during the headache phase. Serotonin, a neurotransmitter released by nerve cells in the brain, is important in controlling blood vessel diameter. Some antimigraine drugs work by blocking the effects of serotonin.

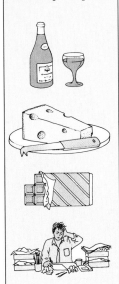

COMMON TRIGGERS OF MIGRAINE ATTACKS

Common triggers include:

◆ Some foods, such as cheese and chocolate (these foods contain chemicals similar to serotonin, a neurotransmitter important in controlling blood vessel diameter, which is involved in migraine.)
◆ Red wine
◆ Stress
◆ Fatigue
◆ Lack of sleep
◆ Some drugs, such as those for angina (chest pain) and the oral contraceptive pill

Variants of migraine

Cluster headaches and paroxysmal hemicrania are uncommon variants of migraine. Their main symptoms are described below. Paroxysmal hemicrania is one-sided headache pain that passes quickly and can occur several times daily. It responds well to the drug indomethacin. Cluster headaches almost always occur in young men. If you suffer from cluster headaches, you should not drink alcohol, because it tends to bring on an attack. Your doctor may prescribe a steroid drug such as prednisone to prevent attacks. Methysergide and lithium carbonate also may be effective. Inhalation of 100 percent oxygen often relieves symptoms of cluster headaches. The drug ergotamine sometimes provides relief but should not be taken for periods longer than 3 weeks or without guidance from your doctor.

CHRONIC TENSION HEADACHES

A constant or recurring headache without nausea, vomiting, or visual disturbance that has occurred intermittently for several months is called a chronic or recurrent tension headache. Doctors once thought muscle contraction around the head and neck, from long-term stress, or depression, caused tension headaches. But recent studies have cast doubt on the role of muscle contraction in these headaches. Authorities now speculate that tension headaches may have causes similar to those of migraine. But recurrent tension headaches usually indicate stress in your life. You should evaluate with your doctor the circumstances that seem to provoke your headaches to see whether they can be reduced or eliminated. Your doctor's reassurance that there is no underlying disease present can help to relieve chronic tension headaches. Brief use of a minor tranquilizer along with a simple analgesic (such as acetaminophen or aspirin) may help break the cycle of recurrent headaches.

Cluster headaches
This disorder typically produces a severe, recurrent headache, watering of one eye, and stuffiness of one nostril, all on one side of the face and head. The pain lasts from 10 minutes to several hours and often awakens the sufferer in the early morning hours. Attacks tend to "cluster," occurring daily for several weeks and then completely clearing, only to return in an additional cluster several months later. Attacks are particularly common in the spring and fall.

Headache affecting one side

Watering eye

Stuffy nostril

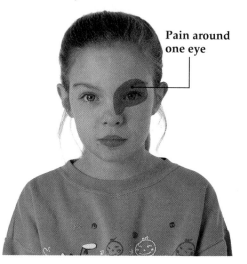

Pain around one eye

Paroxysmal hemicrania
Like a cluster headache, this disorder is a rare variant of migraine. Headaches are one-sided and usually occur around the eye. Attacks are brief, lasting for about 15 minutes. They often occur many times daily.

CASE HISTORY
A WARNING HEADACHE

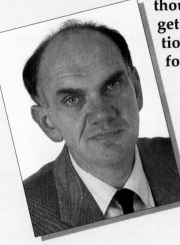

MARLON HAD A KIDNEY TRANSPLANT 2 years ago. During a regular checkup, he mentioned to his doctor that he had had a severe headache the previous day, although he said he did not usually get headaches at all. As a precaution, the doctor referred Marlon for a neurological examination.

PERSONAL DETAILS
Name Marlon Wilson
Age 48
Occupation Taxi driver
Family His father died of kidney failure at 52. His mother is healthy, but takes a beta-blocker for high blood pressure.

MEDICAL BACKGROUND
Ten years ago, Marlon was diagnosed as having polycystic kidneys, a congenital disease (a disease one is born with) in which numerous cysts grow in the kidneys. His kidneys stopped working 2 years ago, and he underwent kidney transplantation. Otherwise, he has been healthy and takes no medication aside from the drugs prescribed to prevent rejection of the transplanted kidney by his body.

THE NEUROLOGICAL CONSULTATION
Marlon's story alerts the neurologist to a potentially serious condition. The doctor tells Marlon that people who have had polycystic kidney disease may also have a small ballooning (aneurysm) in a blood vessel at the base of the brain. The neurologist explains that the aneurysm ruptures in one out of 10 people, releasing blood into the space between the membranes that surround the brain and spinal cord (the subarachnoid space). These hemorrhages generally occur suddenly, resulting in

death before the person reaches the hospital. A few people get a warning headache a week or so before the major hemorrhage. This headache begins when a small amount of blood leaks from the aneurysm.

THE INVESTIGATION
The neurologist arranges for an immediate computed tomography (CT) scan and performs a lumbar puncture to obtain samples of Marlon's cerebrospinal fluid (the fluid that bathes his brain and spinal cord). The CT scan shows no evidence of bleeding, but all samples of cerebrospinal fluid are faintly bloodstained.

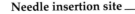
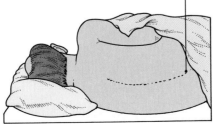

Needle insertion site

THE DIAGNOSIS
The neurologist's diagnosis is SUBARACHNOID HEMORRHAGE, most likely caused by an aneurysm that has begun to leak. He orders immediate carotid angiography, a test in which doctors inject a dye that is visible on X-ray film into the carotid artery, one of the blood vessels that supply the brain. The angiogram shows that Marlon has an aneurysm in the circle of Willis, a collection of arteries at the base of the brain.

THE TREATMENT
Marlon is immediately taken to the operating room, where surgeons place a clip around the base of the aneurysm to stop further bleeding.

THE OUTCOME
Marlon goes home from the hospital without having any disability after 10 days and resumes working 6 weeks later. His doctors say further bleeding is unlikely.

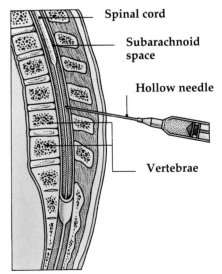

Spinal cord

Subarachnoid space

Hollow needle

Vertebrae

Lumbar puncture
Doctors insert a hollow needle into the subarachnoid space in the lumbar spine. They take samples of cerebrospinal fluid and send them to the laboratory for microscopic and chemical analysis.

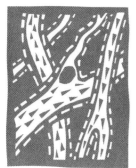

STROKE AND RELATED DISORDERS

EREBROVASCULAR DISEASE (STROKE) can have a devastating effect on its victims and their families. Stroke can cause not only physical impairment but also social isolation and despondency. But rehabilitation programs can return stroke victims to higher levels of functioning. Many stroke victims now lead independent lives.

RISK FACTORS FOR STROKE

The following risk factors increase your chances of a stroke. Most of these can be modified by medical treatment or changes in lifestyle.

◆ Atherosclerosis (narrowing of the arteries)
◆ Uncontrolled hypertension (high blood pressure)
◆ Advanced age
◆ Heart disease (with irregular rhythm)
◆ Polycythemia (increased red blood cell count)
◆ Smoking
◆ Diabetes mellitus
◆ Oral contraceptive use

Each year in the US, stroke occurs in about 100 to 200 people out of 100,000. The number has decreased in the past 50 years, partly because of widespread effective treatment of high blood pressure, the biggest risk factor for strokes. Strokes are uncommon in early and middle life, but their incidence rises steeply with age, particularly after age 65. Stroke is the third leading cause of death in the US, after heart disease and cancer. Most deaths occur in the elderly.

OUTCOME OF STROKES

In about two thirds of people, stroke symptoms are severe enough to warrant hospital admission. Approximately 10 to 25 percent of strokes are fatal. Of the remainder, some cause permanent damage or disability and others have no serious lasting effects, although recovery may not be complete for weeks. Even a mild stroke is a serious warning, because it may herald one or more increasingly severe attacks.

Death rate per 100,000 of the population

Death from stroke
This chart shows the dramatic increase with age in the number of deaths due to stroke. Although the incidence of stroke is greater in men than in women during middle age, more women 75 and older die of strokes, primarily because more women than men survive to this age. These figures are for the US during 1986.

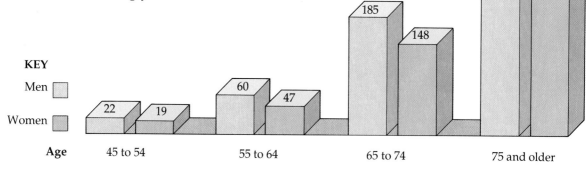

KEY
Men
Women

Age	45 to 54	55 to 64	65 to 74	75 and older
Men	22	60	185	822
Women	19	47	148	868

THE CAUSES OF STROKE

Strokes occur when the blood supply to part of the brain is cut off or when blood leaks into the brain. Interruption of the blood supply damages the brain by depriving it of vital oxygen. Blood leakage impairs the brain by compressing and irritating brain tissue. When nerve cells or tracts in the brain are damaged, they lose their ability to transmit messages to other parts of the body. Important functions, such as thinking, speech, coordination, and motor control, can become impaired. These are the main types of blood vessel disturbance that can lead to stroke:

CEREBRAL HEMORRHAGE

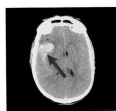

Subarachnoid hemorrhage
This computed tomography (CT) scan shows bleeding on the brain's surface (arrow).

Cerebral hemorrhage occurs when an artery bursts and blood pumps into and damages surrounding brain tissue. A cerebral hemorrhage may take place within the brain tissue (intracerebral) or on the brain's surface (subarachnoid). High blood pressure usually causes intracerebral hemorrhage. Subarachnoid hemorrhage can be caused by an aneurysm or a congenital malformation of blood vessels supplying the brain (see below).

Blockage of tiny vessels
These blockages produce small strokes that occur deep within the brain and may lead to a form of dementia (see page 134). The strokes (called lacunar strokes) result from the blockage of tiny blood vessels that have usually been damaged by years of hypertension (high blood pressure) or diabetes.

Cerebral artery thrombosis
Cerebral artery thrombosis occurs when one of the arteries to the brain is blocked by a blood clot. The blockage usually builds up because of atherosclerosis, the narrowing of arteries by fatty deposits (called atheroma). When oxygen cannot reach the brain, tissue in the area of brain supplied by that artery quickly dies.

Cerebral embolism
Cerebral embolism is another form of arterial blockage, occurring when an embolus, a piece of fat or clotted blood (or some air), that has traveled from elsewhere in the body, lodges in the artery. The embolus is often a blood clot that circulates through the bloodstream from an atherosclerotic artery or from a diseased heart until it wedges in a vessel.

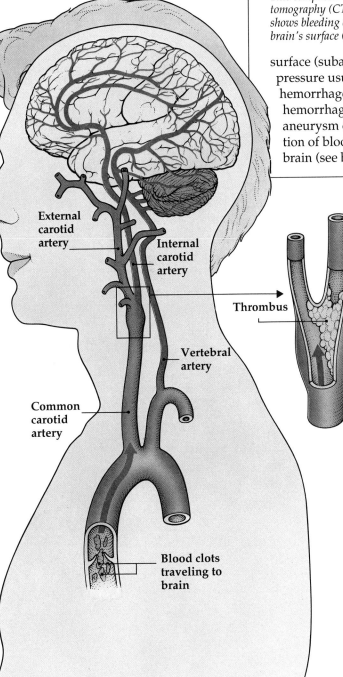

External carotid artery

Internal carotid artery

Vertebral artery

Common carotid artery

Blood clots traveling to brain

Thrombus

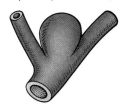

Aneurysm
A weak spot in an artery wall can expand like a balloon, forming an aneurysm (bulge in the artery wall). It may rupture spontaneously.

Arteriovenous malformation
Some people are born with a tangled mass of blood vessels in a part of the brain. There, arteries and veins have fewer capillary connections than normal. Pressure elevates and blood may leak into the brain.

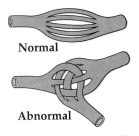

Normal

Abnormal

WHAT TO DO

If you are with someone who you think may have had a stroke:

◆ Get immediate medical attention
◆ Loosen any tight clothing
◆ Do not administer anything by mouth
◆ Place the person in a comfortable reclining position

SYMPTOMS AND SIGNS

A stroke happens when the brain's blood supply becomes disrupted. This disruption interferes with the sensory, motor, or mental functions of the brain. The symptoms and signs of stroke depend on which part of the brain is affected. For example, if the area that controls language (usually on the left side of the brain) is affected, speech difficulties arise. Damage to the brain stem and cerebellum, which are major body control centers, cause problems with muscular coordination, swallowing, and eye movements. Symptoms usually develop over minutes or hours but occasionally evolve over several days. Only one side of the body is affected in many cases, because usually only one side of the brain is damaged. Each side of the body is controlled by the opposite side of the cerebral cortex, so symptoms often occur on the opposite side of the body from the damaged side of the brain.

A COMMON SITE OF STROKE: THE LEFT MIDDLE CEREBRAL ARTERY

The area of the brain supplied by the middle cerebral artery is the region where strokes most commonly strike. If the left middle cerebral artery is blocked, disturbance of speech and other language skills may occur; speech is usually not affected by strokes caused by blockage of the right middle cerebral artery. The regions of the cerebrum damaged by a major stroke and their corresponding symptoms and signs are listed below.

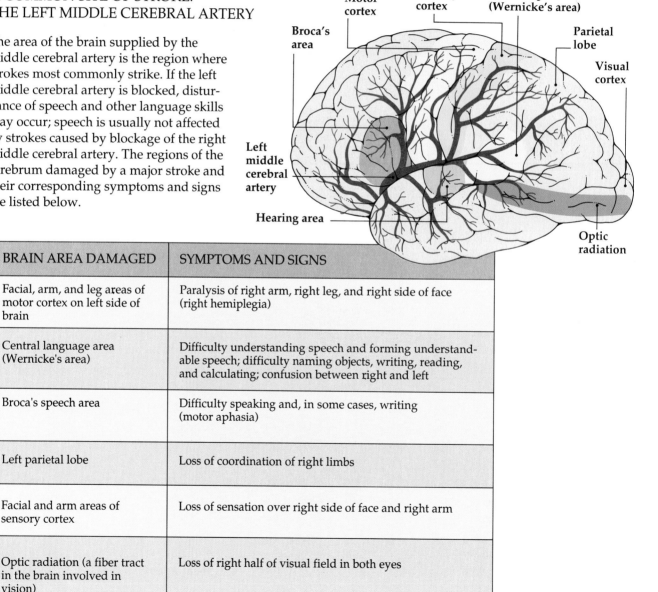

BRAIN AREA DAMAGED	SYMPTOMS AND SIGNS
Facial, arm, and leg areas of motor cortex on left side of brain	Paralysis of right arm, right leg, and right side of face (right hemiplegia)
Central language area (Wernicke's area)	Difficulty understanding speech and forming understandable speech; difficulty naming objects, writing, reading, and calculating; confusion between right and left
Broca's speech area	Difficulty speaking and, in some cases, writing (motor aphasia)
Left parietal lobe	Loss of coordination of right limbs
Facial and arm areas of sensory cortex	Loss of sensation over right side of face and right arm
Optic radiation (a fiber tract in the brain involved in vision)	Loss of right half of visual field in both eyes

TRANSIENT ISCHEMIC ATTACK

A transient ischemic attack (TIA) is a brief loss of brain function that resembles a stroke. TIAs usually last only 10 to 30 minutes but may last 24 hours. TIAs are important warning signals that the person has an increased risk for stroke. About 8 to 12 percent of people who have TIAs will have a stroke in the following year if the attacks are not treated.

What are the symptoms?

The symptoms of a TIA resemble those of a stroke but usually are more limited. They occur suddenly, last only a short time, and then disappear. Symptoms vary depending on the part of the brain that is affected but commonly include weakness, clumsiness, or numbness confined to one side of the body or one arm or leg. Visual loss or double vision, speech impairment, and difficulty reading or understanding speech may also occur. Although complete recovery follows a TIA, the attacks may recur.

What is the treatment?

If you have had a TIA and your life-style increases your chances of stroke (for example, if you smoke or have high blood pressure), your doctor will advise you about ways to reduce your risk.

Your doctor may also ask you to take 50 to 300 milligrams of aspirin every day, or every other day, for the rest of your life. Research has shown that aspirin is effective in reducing the chances of stroke following TIAs. Aspirin helps to prevent recurrent attacks by reducing the likelihood of blood clot formation. Other, more powerful anticoagulant drugs (those that reduce blood clots) may also be prescribed.

If the attack was caused by a narrowed artery, doctors may perform surgery to remove the fatty deposits (atheroma) that caused the narrowing and led to the TIA.

WHAT CAUSES A TIA?

Just as a permanently blocked artery in the brain causes stroke, a narrowed or temporarily blocked artery in the brain brings about a TIA. The usual obstruction is a clump of blood or other material that temporarily impedes blood flow, producing strokelike symptoms until the blockage is dispersed and carried away.

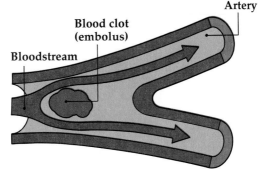

Embolus
A small clot of blood particles (embolus) carried in the bloodstream from elsewhere in the body settles into an artery that supplies the brain.

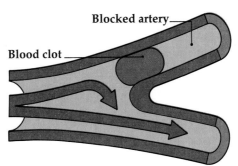

Blockage
The clot blocks the artery, impeding the flow of blood to an area of the brain and thereby depriving it of needed oxygen.

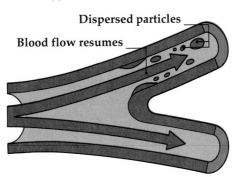

Restored blood flow
The clot of blood particles becomes dispersed and swept away, circulation to the deprived tissues resumes, and the symptoms disappear.

WARNING

A TIA may herald a major stroke. As many as one third of people with TIAs will have a stroke within 5 years if they are not treated. These people also carry an increased risk for heart attacks. If you suspect that you have had a TIA, consult your doctor immediately. He or she will perform a series of tests that may include cerebral angiography or ultrasound studies to investigate the carotid artery in the neck (see page 111). Once your doctor establishes the exact cause of the TIA, he or she will discuss treatment with you and your family.

MONITOR YOUR SYMPTOMS
DIZZINESS

Dizziness, a sensation that you or your surroundings are moving or spinning, can commonly arise following a head injury. If you become dizzy after injuring your head, you should seek medical care immediately. Dizziness, unsteadiness, or the feeling of being out of balance, that occurs without obvious explanation, may be a symptom of another underlying medical disorder.

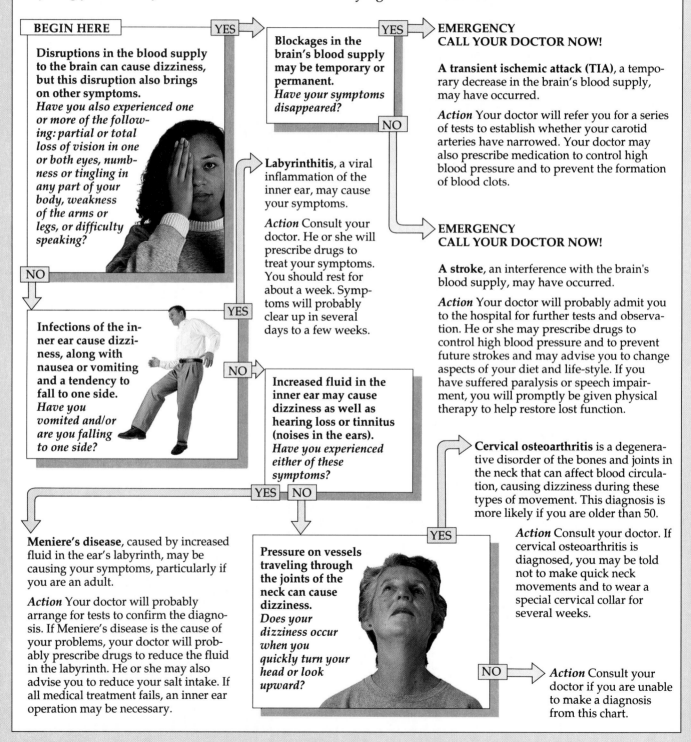

BEGIN HERE ── YES ──▶

Disruptions in the blood supply to the brain can cause dizziness, but this disruption also brings on other symptoms.
Have you also experienced one or more of the following: partial or total loss of vision in one or both eyes, numbness or tingling in any part of your body, weakness of the arms or legs, or difficulty speaking?

NO ▼

Infections of the inner ear cause dizziness, along with nausea or vomiting and a tendency to fall to one side.
Have you vomited and/or are you falling to one side?

── YES ──▶

── NO ──▶

Blockages in the brain's blood supply may be temporary or permanent.
Have your symptoms disappeared?

── YES ──▶

NO ▼

Labyrinthitis, a viral inflammation of the inner ear, may cause your symptoms.

Action Consult your doctor. He or she will prescribe drugs to treat your symptoms. You should rest for about a week. Symptoms will probably clear up in several days to a few weeks.

Increased fluid in the inner ear may cause dizziness as well as hearing loss or tinnitus (noises in the ears).
Have you experienced either of these symptoms?

YES │ NO ▼

**EMERGENCY
CALL YOUR DOCTOR NOW!**

A transient ischemic attack (TIA), a temporary decrease in the brain's blood supply, may have occurred.

Action Your doctor will refer you for a series of tests to establish whether your carotid arteries have narrowed. Your doctor may also prescribe medication to control high blood pressure and to prevent the formation of blood clots.

**EMERGENCY
CALL YOUR DOCTOR NOW!**

A stroke, an interference with the brain's blood supply, may have occurred.

Action Your doctor will probably admit you to the hospital for further tests and observation. He or she may prescribe drugs to control high blood pressure and to prevent future strokes and may advise you to change aspects of your diet and life-style. If you have suffered paralysis or speech impairment, you will promptly be given physical therapy to help restore lost function.

Cervical osteoarthritis is a degenerative disorder of the bones and joints in the neck that can affect blood circulation, causing dizziness during these types of movement. This diagnosis is more likely if you are older than 50.

Action Consult your doctor. If cervical osteoarthritis is diagnosed, you may be told not to make quick neck movements and to wear a special cervical collar for several weeks.

Meniere's disease, caused by increased fluid in the ear's labyrinth, may be causing your symptoms, particularly if you are an adult.

Action Your doctor will probably arrange for tests to confirm the diagnosis. If Meniere's disease is the cause of your problems, your doctor will probably prescribe drugs to reduce the fluid in the labyrinth. He or she may also advise you to reduce your salt intake. If all medical treatment fails, an inner ear operation may be necessary.

Pressure on vessels traveling through the joints of the neck can cause dizziness.
Does your dizziness occur when you quickly turn your head or look upward?

── YES ──▶

NO ──▶ *Action* Consult your doctor if you are unable to make a diagnosis from this chart.

DIAGNOSIS

A doctor can usually diagnose a stroke fairly rapidly based on an account of events from the person or a witness or following an examination of the person. It is important for the doctor to rule out other causes of the sudden onset of symptoms. Sometimes a tumor or infection can cause symptoms similar to those of a stroke.

Imaging techniques

Computed tomography (CT) scanning of the brain can help identify the cause of a stroke or TIA. CT scans can reveal aneurysms, the site of intracerebral bleeding, and, within a few days, areas of brain damaged by oxygen deprivation (ischemia). CT scanning can distinguish strokes caused by blockage from those caused by bleeding (hemorrhage).

CT scanning can also differentiate symptoms caused by stroke from those caused by another disorder, such as a brain tumor, brain abscess, subdural hemorrhage, or encephalitis (inflammation of the brain). CT scanning is usually the first imaging technique doctors use.

Magnetic resonance imaging (MRI) can be used to identify the precise location of a stroke, especially if the problem is in the back portion of the brain. MRI is especially valuable in detecting disorders in the white matter of the brain, such as multiple sclerosis and some types of brain tumors.

Carotid artery angiogram
The image at right shows a narrowing of the internal carotid artery in the neck (arrow).

OTHER TESTS

Doctors perform lumbar puncture to identify blood in the cerebrospinal fluid, which indicates hemorrhage. Electroencephalograms can reveal marked abnormalities in the brain's electrical activity but have limited diagnostic value in the investigation of stroke. Doctors perform blood tests to check for any abnormalities that may contribute to a stroke. Electrocardiography and echocardiography detect underlying abnormalities in heart rhythm or blood clots in the upper heart chamber.

CT scan
The large white area on this scan defines a hemorrhage (bleeding area) within the brain.

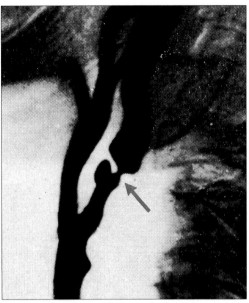

Investigating blood flow

Cerebral angiography can identify sites of blood vessel narrowing or obstruction that may be causing stroke or TIA. This procedure does involve some risk, so it is performed only if the cause of the stroke can be treated with surgery (for example, if the stroke has been caused by blood vessel malformation or blockage in the neck vessels). Digital subtraction angiography, in which a computer processes images to remove background information, is somewhat safer but may produce less clear images.

Doctors now use a number of ultrasound techniques that are based on detection and computer analysis of reflected echoes from sound waves passed through the body to investigate blood flow. These techniques can determine the degree of narrowing of the carotid arteries in the neck. Doctors also use such sonar ultrasound techniques to investigate the blood flow in the carotid arteries in a suspected TIA.

TREATMENT OF ACUTE STAGES OF STROKE

To treat the initial or acute stage of a stroke, doctors first perform any lifesaving procedures necessary to maintain the person's breathing and circu-

SURGICAL PROCEDURES
CLIPPING AN ANEURYSM

S UBARACHNOID HEMORRHAGE **(bleeding into the space between the membranes that surround the brain and spinal cord) most often results from a ruptured berry aneurysm, a small berry-shaped swelling in a blood vessel. Neurosurgeons can prevent further bleeding by placing a metal clip around the neck of the aneurysm, closing it off and isolating it from the rest of the artery.**

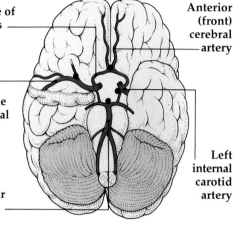

Circle of Willis

Anterior (front) cerebral artery

Middle cerebral artery

Left internal carotid artery

Basilar artery

Aneurysm sites
Most aneurysms in the brain occur in the collection of arteries at the base of the brain (the circle of Willis), particularly at the points where the arteries divide into two or more branches. The illustration at left shows the most common sites (black spots) of aneurysms (the brain is viewed from below and part of the temporal lobe has been cut away).

REPAIRING A RUPTURED BERRY ANEURYSM

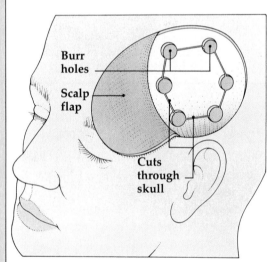

Burr holes

Scalp flap

Cuts through skull

1 Under general anesthesia, the patient undergoes craniotomy (removal or opening of part of the skull). First, the surgical team shaves an area of the scalp and cuts away the layers of skin, muscle, and membrane at the surgical site. Then they drill burr holes in the skull and cut between the holes with a flexible, sawtooth wire.

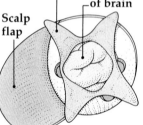

Membranes covering brain

Surface of brain

Scalp flap

2 The surgeon lifts back the lid of bone on a hinge of muscle or removes it completely. The membranes covering the brain are then opened, allowing access to the brain.

3 The neurosurgeon uses a binocular operating microscope to magnify the aneurysm and the artery in which it occurs. He or she carefully separates the neck of the aneurysm from the surrounding tissues.

4 When the neck of the aneurysm is entirely visible, the neurosurgeon places a small metal clip across it, isolating the aneurysm from the circulation. The neurosurgeon then replaces the lid of bone and closes the patient's skull.

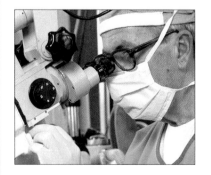

Berry aneurysm

Clip

lation. When the person stabilizes, doctors evaluate the severity of the stroke.

In the hospital, nurses give the continuous care needed to prevent pressure sores, limb contractures (stiffening), pneumonia, and loss of morale. This therapy often includes passive exercise of the weakened limb or limbs. Drowsy or comatose stroke victims require intravenous feeding, and those who have difficulty swallowing may need to be fed by means of a tube inserted into the nose. Temporary drainage of the bladder via a catheter may be required for stroke victims who have lost bladder control.

Drug treatment

Doctors sometimes prescribe diuretic drugs (such as mannitol), which expel excess water, to reduce brain swelling, especially for hemorrhages inside the skull. Small doses of aspirin may help prevent recurrences in a person whose stroke was caused by an embolism. Anticoagulant drugs, which inhibit blood clotting, may be used as well (see above right). Research is under way to evaluate the use of tissue plasminogen activator and other clot-dissolving drugs to treat stroke from arterial blockage.

Surgical treatment

Surgery on affected blood vessels can reduce the risk of another stroke. Carotid endarterectomy is a surgical procedure that removes the blockage from certain parts of the carotid artery. This procedure may be recommended for people who suffer from transient ischemic attacks. (See page 112 for a description of surgical treatment for subarachnoid hemorrhage from a ruptured berry aneurysm.)

REHABILITATION AFTER A STROKE

The best form of treatment for stroke is a rehabilitation program that fulfills the stroke victim's physical, social, and

ANTICOAGULANT DRUGS

Anticoagulant drugs, such as heparin, inhibit the clotting of blood. Doctors often give anticoagulant drugs when they are certain the thrombus is in the heart. In other cases, anticoagulant drugs may be dangerous because of the risk of bleeding into the brain. These drugs block the action of certain blood-clotting factors that convert fibrinogen into fibrin, the protein that binds platelets into blood clots (see below).

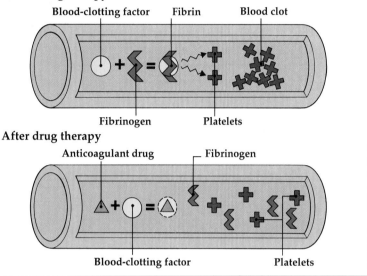

Before drug therapy

Blood-clotting factor   Fibrin   Blood clot

Fibrinogen   Platelets

After drug therapy

Anticoagulant drug   Fibrinogen

Blood-clotting factor   Platelets

emotional needs. Rehabilitation must begin without delay after a stroke to ensure the best chances for recovery. A team of professionals in nursing; physical, speech, and occupational therapy; and social work often pool their skills to give stroke victims comprehensive treatment. Rehabilitation programs usually begin in the hospital and continue at an outpatient clinic or at home.

Physical therapy is the mainstay of rehabilitation. The physical therapist teaches stroke victims exercises to retrain muscles and restore as much function as possible to the affected part of the body. Physical therapy can also help the stroke victim learn how to compensate for his or her disability. For example, a person who has lost the use of a leg can learn to make more effective use of the other leg and the arms.

One of the most important factors in successful recovery is the person's own

ADAPTIVE AIDS

Stroke victims can compensate for their disabilities by using special adaptive aids, such as a wall-mounted device for taking off screw caps, or a long clasper for reaching higher shelves. Handrails at the sides of the toilet and the bathtub help the stroke victim maintain balance while transferring from a wheelchair. A telephone that has a loudspeaker and amplifier can be used to speak and hear from a distance.

ASK YOUR DOCTOR
STROKE

Q **I've been having periods of blindness in my right eye that are similar to a curtain falling from top to bottom. It lasts only a few seconds. Should I be worried?**

A See your doctor immediately. The episodes you describe are typical of a condition called amaurosis fugax and suggest you may be having transient ischemic attacks, temporary losses of blood supply, in the retina of your eye. The main blood vessel that supplies large portions of the brain also supplies this part of the eye.

Q **I often get a headache on the right side of my head, less often on the left, that is preceded by flashing lights in front of my eyes. I often feel sick with the headache. Am I about to have a stroke?**

A If you have no other risk factors for stroke in your medical history and your doctor finds no signs to suggest stroke during an examination, you probably are not at risk for stroke. Your symptoms sound much like migraine. But you should have your blood pressure checked as a precaution.

Q **My father, grandfather, and paternal aunt all died of a stroke. Is stroke hereditary? What can I do to prevent it?**

A There are several types of strokes with different causes. Most are not hereditary. Talk to your doctor, who will review your family history. High blood pressure is a risk factor for stroke and hypertension does run in families. You can cut your risk for all types of stroke by eating a low-fat, low-salt diet and exercising regularly. Don't smoke. Keep your weight down.

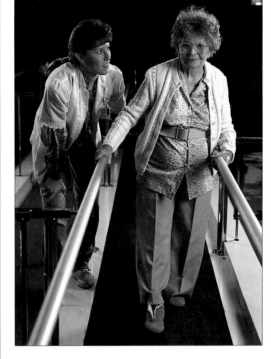

Learning to walk again
A physical therapist teaches a stroke victim exercises to retrain muscles. The person may progress from using parallel bars, to walking with a cane or a walker, and eventually to walking without help.

motivation. Stroke victims must work hard to regain lost function. Persistence may be difficult when the person understandably feels depressed or negative. The support, patience, and encouragement from relatives and friends is key in improving the person's mental attitude.

More than 80 percent of stroke survivors eventually learn to walk again. About two thirds of these people are able to live alone and manage their own lives.

Occupational therapy
People who have had strokes may require occupational therapy to help them relearn muscular control and coordination. Such therapy helps them cope with everyday tasks, such as dressing, bathing, and cooking.

SPEECH THERAPY

Speech therapy after a stroke retrains vocalization, pronunciation, and other language skills. Speech therapists can also help with the swallowing problems that sometimes occur. The speech therapist may explain the stroke victim's problems to other members of the family and teach them to help.

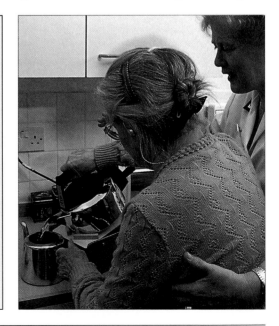

CASE HISTORY
SUDDEN LOSS OF SENSATION

J OANNA HAS SMOKED HEAVILY **and has been overweight all her adult life. She has been careless about taking her high blood pressure medication. One morning, Joanna had difficulty getting out of bed. Her left arm hung limp and her left leg would not support her. She struggled to the phone and called an ambulance to take her to the hospital.**

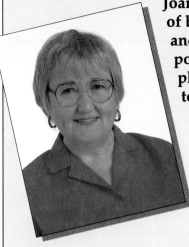

PERSONAL DETAILS
Name Joanna Van der Wall
Age 62
Occupation Homemaker
Family Joanna is a widow and has no children. Her father lived to be 92.

MEDICAL BACKGROUND
Joanna suffers from hypertension (high blood pressure) but has repeatedly ignored her doctor's advice to quit smoking and to lose weight. She stubbornly believes that she will live as long as her father and not become seriously ill. She also admits to skipping her medication. Recently, Joanna has experienced short episodes of partial vision loss in her right eye. Her doctor has told her these are transient ischemic attacks that should be investigated by a neurologist. Joanna has ignored his advice.

THE INVESTIGATIONS
When Joanna arrives in the emergency room, she still can't move her left arm. Sensation is reduced on her left side and she can't see things in her left field of vision. A computed tomography (CT) scan shows that an area on the right side of her brain near the surface appears to have been deprived of its blood supply. The doctors perform a test called a carotid Doppler study, which shows that Joanna's right internal carotid

artery is completely blocked. They conclude that Joanna has probably suffered a cerebral thrombosis (blockage) of an artery in the brain.

THE DIAGNOSIS
The doctors admit Joanna to the hospital and monitor her closely. Her leg weakness begins to subside the second day, but her arm remains paralyzed. Joanna's doctors tell her she has suffered a STROKE.

THE TREATMENT
Joanna begins a program of physical therapy in the hospital. She regains enough control of

Continued improvement
Following her physical and occupational therapy program, Joanna occasionally returns to her physical therapist to plan additional exercises.

her leg to begin doing exercises on her own. She eventually progresses to the parallel bars, where she relearns how to walk with her left leg in a brace. Joanna also attends the hospital's occupational therapy classes. These classes help her master the skills needed for activities of everyday living, such as dressing and bathing, with her right arm only. She also learns how to cook with special devices. After 3 weeks in the hospital, Joanna transfers to a rehabilitation hospital to complete her recovery. During the next 4 weeks, Joanna's condition steadily improves. With help and encouragement from the health care team, and her own determination, Joanna is eventually able to walk, but her left arm moves only slightly. Joanna's vision is still impaired on the left side, but she learns to compensate.

THE OUTCOME
Since her stroke, Joanna has not smoked a single cigarette. She has lost 40 pounds and has kept her weight down to this level. At her doctor's suggestion, she learns to measure her own blood pressure weekly using an electronic monitoring device. She takes her medication and sees her doctor regularly.

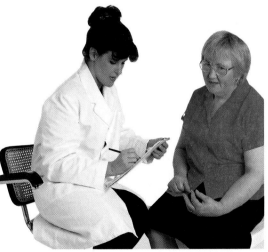

PARKINSON'S DISEASE

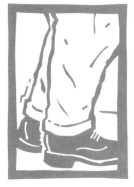

PARKINSON'S DISEASE occasionally occurs in young people but mainly affects people older than 60. With today's treatment, people affected by the disease can obtain considerable relief of symptoms and live, on average, almost as long as unaffected people of the same age.

Parkinson's disease, a brain disorder that causes muscle tremor, stiffness, and weakness, occurs in approximately one person per 1,000 worldwide, increasing to one per 200 among people older than 60. In the US, 50,000 new cases occur every year. The incidence of Parkinson's disease is slightly higher among men and is lower among smokers, although doctors do not know why. The cause of Parkinson's disease remains unknown. Presently no cure exists but treatment can minimize symptoms. Exercise, special aids in the home, and encouragement from family and friends can do much to improve morale and mobility.

WHAT IS PARKINSON'S DISEASE?

Parkinson's disease has probably existed for centuries, but it was first recognized as a separate condition in 1817 when the English doctor James Parkinson published *An Essay on the Shaking Palsy*. The patients he described were suffering from a central nervous system disorder that affected movement and speech.

The symptoms of Parkinson's disease arise from the progressive degeneration of cells, especially in a small area of the brain called the substantia nigra (see page

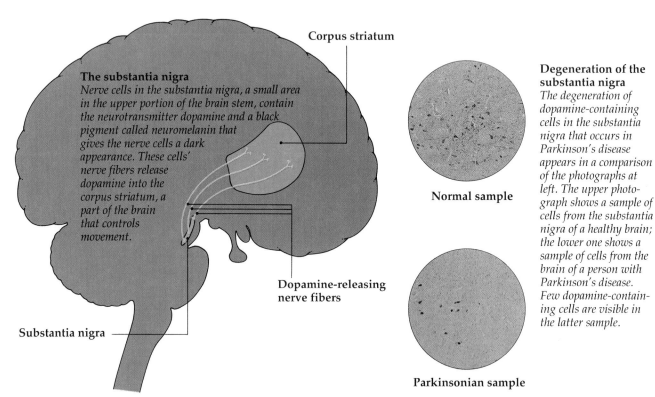

The substantia nigra
Nerve cells in the substantia nigra, a small area in the upper portion of the brain stem, contain the neurotransmitter dopamine and a black pigment called neuromelanin that gives the nerve cells a dark appearance. These cells' nerve fibers release dopamine into the corpus striatum, a part of the brain that controls movement.

Corpus striatum

Dopamine-releasing nerve fibers

Substantia nigra

Normal sample

Parkinsonian sample

Degeneration of the substantia nigra
The degeneration of dopamine-containing cells in the substantia nigra that occurs in Parkinson's disease appears in a comparison of the photographs at left. The upper photograph shows a sample of cells from the substantia nigra of a healthy brain; the lower one shows a sample of cells from the brain of a person with Parkinson's disease. Few dopamine-containing cells are visible in the latter sample.

WHY DOES PARKINSON'S DISEASE AFFECT MOVEMENT?

In Parkinson's disease, damage to the cells in the substantia nigra affects the muscle-coordinating function of the basal ganglia, located deep within the cerebrum and the upper brain stem (see page 53). The damage also disrupts the balance between dopamine and acetylcholine, neurotransmitters involved in the control of movement. The difference between the healthy and diseased states is shown here.

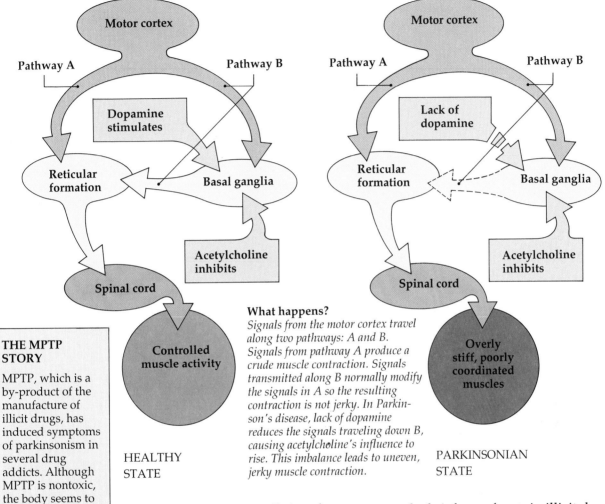

What happens?
Signals from the motor cortex travel along two pathways: A and B. Signals from pathway A produce a crude muscle contraction. Signals transmitted along B normally modify the signals in A so the resulting contraction is not jerky. In Parkinson's disease, lack of dopamine reduces the signals traveling down B, causing acetylcholine's influence to rise. This imbalance leads to uneven, jerky muscle contraction.

HEALTHY STATE

PARKINSONIAN STATE

THE MPTP STORY

MPTP, which is a by-product of the manufacture of illicit drugs, has induced symptoms of parkinsonism in several drug addicts. Although MPTP is nontoxic, the body seems to convert it into a highly toxic substance that attacks substantia nigra cells. These findings suggest that an environmental toxin, possibly related to MPTP, may contribute to naturally occurring Parkinson's disease. The findings have also spurred further study of drugs for parkinsonism.

116), although nerve cells in other areas of the brain may also degenerate. This degeneration leads to a lack of dopamine, a neurotransmitter that is vital to the normal control of movement. The reason for this deterioration remains unknown, although drugs, toxins, or infections known to alter dopamine production or activity can sometimes produce identical symptoms. In cases such as these, a person is said to be suffering from parkinsonism. For example, short-term treatment with antipsychotic drugs, carbon monoxide poisoning, the rare brain infection encephalitis lethargica, or the brief use of certain illicit drugs of abuse can produce symptoms of parkinsonism in people.

The search for a cause

Although two members of a family may develop Parkinson's disease, no evidence exists that the disease is inherited. This fact has led biochemical researchers to look for an environmental cause, such as a virus, a toxic chemical, or an imbalance of essential minerals. No environmental cause has yet been discovered, but some evidence suggests that environmental factors may play a role.

WHAT ARE THE SYMPTOMS?

The symptoms of Parkinson's disease fall into four groups: tremor, slowness of voluntary movement, muscle stiffness (rigidity), and postural changes. Slowing of movement may restrict speech and facial mobility, giving some sufferers an expressionless appearance.

Parkinson's disease affects different people in various ways. Some sufferers experience only a few symptoms, particularly in the early phase of the illness. Certain people exhibit tremor as their dominant symptom, while others only experience clumsiness and some stiffness in one hand. The onset of symptoms is often asymmetrical, affecting one side of the body more than the other.

Parkinson's disease is progressive, which means symptoms get worse as time goes on. In its advanced stages, the disease can be extremely disabling, producing severe weakness. The onset of the disease is subtle, so early symptoms may not be detected by the sufferer or his or her doctor. Symptoms are often mistaken for signs of aging or depression.

There are no specific tests that can aid in the diagnosis of Parkinson's disease. Doctors usually diagnose the disease based on the person's symptoms and physical examination findings. When the diagnosis is in doubt, during the early phases, doctors sometimes adopt a "wait-and-see" approach.

MENTAL EFFECTS

Parkinson's disease does not impair intellect in its early stages but may do so late in the course of the illness. Dementia among Parkinson's disease sufferers, which more often affects older patients, sometimes results from coexisting Alzheimer's disease (senile dementia).

Postural signs
As Parkinson's disease progresses, posture becomes increasingly stooped. The person tends to bend the trunk forward and often has difficulty maintaining his or her balance. As the person moves forward, he or she often takes small, shuffling steps and sometimes accelerates to an increasingly rapid walking pace to avoid falling.

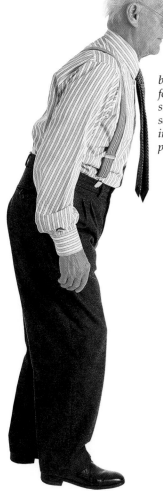

Tremor
Hand tremor is an early manifestation of Parkinson's disease. Initially, tremor often affects only one hand and improves or disappears when the person performs purposeful movement. Tremor later spreads to involve the head, jaws, and legs.

Small handwriting
Very small handwriting (micrographia) that shows signs of tremor is a hallmark of Parkinson's disease. Legibility often improves with drug treatment.

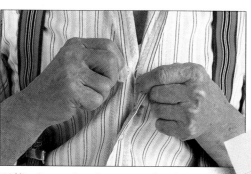

Difficulty performing manual tasks
Slowness of movement, tremor, and muscle rigidity from Parkinson's disease make it increasingly difficult for sufferers to perform manual tasks, such as writing or dressing.

DRUG TREATMENT

Although brain cell degeneration in Parkinson's disease cannot be stopped, antiparkinson drugs minimize the symptoms for many years. Treatment attempts to restore the balance between dopamine and acetylcholine to as normal a level as possible, as shown at right. Various drugs or drug combinations accomplish this goal.

Before the dopamine-boosting drug levodopa became widely available in the late 1960s, anticholinergic drugs were the principal drugs used to treat Parkinson's disease. Today, levodopa, the most commonly prescribed antiparkinson drug, provides considerable benefit for several years. Combining a reduced dosage of levodopa with a drug called carbidopa decreases gastrointestinal side effects. Eventually, symptoms begin to reappear due to severe progression of the underlying disease.

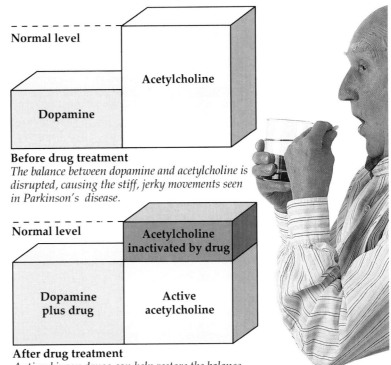

Before drug treatment
The balance between dopamine and acetylcholine is disrupted, causing the stiff, jerky movements seen in Parkinson's disease.

After drug treatment
Antiparkinson drugs can help restore the balance between dopamine and acetylcholine, although never to normal levels, by boosting dopamine levels or inactivating some acetylcholine. Treatment often combines the two approaches.

TYPE	ACTION	COMMENTS
ANTICHOLINERGIC DRUGS **Examples:** benztropine, orphenadrine, procyclidine	Interfere with the action of acetylcholine on brain cells and reduce its relative overactivity in Parkinson's disease.	Effective in early disease stages when symptoms are mild. Most appropriate for younger patients, because treatment may lead to confusion and impaired memory in elderly patients.
DOPAMINE-BOOSTING DRUGS **Examples:** levodopa, levodopa-carbidopa	Absorbed through the digestive tract into the bloodstream and converted to dopamine in the brain to help restore dopamine levels.	Usually prescribed when anticholinergic drug activity begins to weaken. The combination of levodopa-carbidopa works best because carbidopa prevents levodopa from being used up before it reaches the brain. Side effects include nausea, vomiting, and flushing. A reaction known as the "on-off" syndrome sometimes develops after long-term treatment.
DOPAMINE AGONISTS **Examples:** bromocriptine, pergolide	Amplify the effects of dopamine by mimicking its natural activity.	May cause nausea, vomiting, and decreased blood pressure. Often used when the effectiveness of dopamine-boosting drugs wanes.
DOPAMINE-RELEASING DRUGS **Example:** amantadine	Boost dopamine activity by mobilizing dopamine without replenishing the deficiency.	Relieve symptoms in mild cases of Parkinson's disease and have few side effects. Effectiveness weakens after a few months.
MONOAMINE OXIDASE B INHIBITORS **Example:** selegiline	Halt disease progression by inhibiting the enzyme monoamine oxidase B. This enzyme plays a role in converting MPTP (see page 117) into a neurotoxin.	May stop cell degeneration if disease is caused, even in part, by a toxin similar to MPTP. Further research must confirm this theory.

OTHER TREATMENTS

Clinical trials have involved neurosurgical implantation or injection of tissue or cells into the brain to replace areas damaged by Parkinson's disease. The implanted tissue comes from the patient's adrenal gland, as shown at right.

Such transplantations are not yet widely performed. Considered experimental, these operations produce inconsistent results of variable duration. Controversy surrounds a technique, called fetal tissue transplant, that uses cells from the substantia nigra of aborted fetuses. Nevertheless, such techniques hold the possibility of effective future treatment.

COPING WITH PARKINSON'S DISEASE

Coming to terms with a diagnosis of Parkinson's disease can be very difficult because of restrictions the disease imposes. Mental and physical activity make coping with the symptoms easier, but the attitudes of others toward the condition can create problems. For example, overly helpful relatives may rush to perform tasks that the person with Parkinson's disease finds difficult. Slow speech may give a false impression of slow mental activity. These perceptions may encourage the person to become inactive and apathetic.

Depression is a common and natural reaction to the diagnosis of any chronic disease. In some cases, depression seems to be part of the illness and may even predate more obvious symptoms. In addition, antiparkinson drugs sometimes have a depressant effect.

Outside interests often help to lift depression. But feelings of depression should be discussed with a doctor because treatment with antidepressant drugs may aid in recovery. Joining a support group for persons with Parkinson's disease may improve morale.

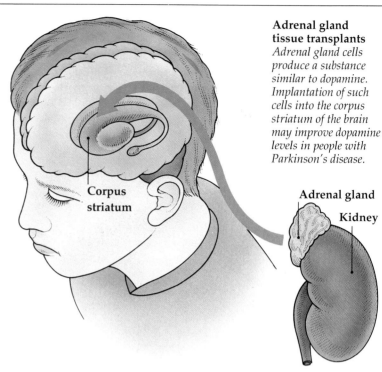

Adrenal gland tissue transplants
Adrenal gland cells produce a substance similar to dopamine. Implantation of such cells into the corpus striatum of the brain may improve dopamine levels in people with Parkinson's disease.

Corpus striatum

Adrenal gland

Kidney

STAYING ACTIVE

A regular exercise routine and general activity can help control the symptoms of Parkinson's disease. Sufferers should obtain guidelines from a doctor to develop a suitable program of home exercise, perhaps along with physical therapy. One of the easiest and most beneficial forms of exercise is regular walking. To realize the full benefits of a walking program, people with Parkinson's disease should follow the suggestions below:

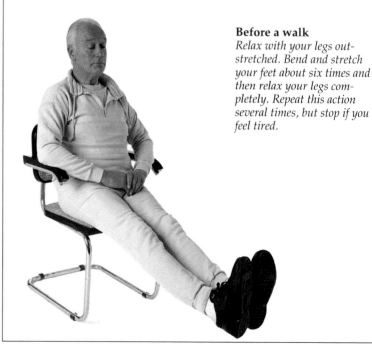

Before a walk
Relax with your legs outstretched. Bend and stretch your feet about six times and then relax your legs completely. Repeat this action several times, but stop if you feel tired.

General health

To minimize Parkinson's disease symptoms, the person should maintain a healthy life-style. His or her surroundings should be kept cheerful and friends and family should provide encouragement to keep morale high. Coughs, flu, or an upset stomach may aggravate movement problems and should be reported to a doctor.

Many people who have Parkinson's disease do not require a special diet. Because the disease tends to cause constipation, increased dietary fiber, from whole grains and fresh fruits and vegetables, may be helpful. Ample fluid intake will also help the person avoid constipation. Parkinson's disease can cause weight loss, so sufferers sometimes receive special dietary supplements.

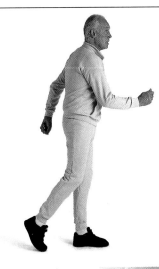

During a walk
Steer clear of crowded places to avoid the anxiety of feeling rushed. Develop a steady rhythm in your walking stride, remembering to strike the ground with the heel first. Try to maintain a relaxed, upright posture and avoid bending your trunk forward. Walk as far as you can without becoming fatigued.

Lengthening your stride
Trace a series of lines on the floor as far apart as you can comfortably reach with each step. Practice walking with an even stride, using the marks as a guide. Try to increase your stride each week.

ASK YOUR DOCTOR PARKINSON'S DISEASE

Q Why haven't any of the drugs prescribed for Parkinson's disease helped me?

A There are three possible reasons. First, you may not have taken the most effective drugs available. Second, the dose may have been too low. Increased dosage under medical supervision may improve your symptoms. Finally, you may have one of a group of rare conditions that sometimes mimic Parkinson's disease. Ask your doctor to reevaluate your current treatment and, if necessary, to refer you to a neurologist who specializes in movement disorders.

Q Is it possible that my children or grandchildren could inherit my Parkinson's disease?

A There is no evidence to suggest that Parkinson's disease is hereditary, although more than one person in a family may be affected.

Q I have a tremor that affects both my hands, but I am otherwise healthy. Is this a sign of Parkinson's disease?

A Probably not. Many people have a physiological tremor that appears during times of stress, hunger, or fatigue. Some people have a persistent tremor that may be inherited. Both types can be seen in the outstretched arm, unlike the parkinsonian tremor, which often occurs when the arm is relaxed. Both of these tremors are benign conditions that will not lead to Parkinson's disease. Your tremor may be suppressed with drug treatment.

HEAD AND NECK INJURY

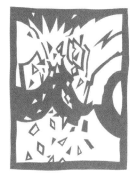

I F YOU RECEIVE a blow to your head – as the result of an athletic activity or in an accident at work, on the road, or at home – when is it dangerous? When should you seek medical care? Most of us have bumped our heads or have had a more serious head injury, whether it was to the scalp, skull, or brain. Head injuries that affect the brain are the most serious. But many other types of head injuries can also have serious consequences.

The most obviously dangerous head injuries are those that penetrate both the scalp and skull, damaging the brain. Such injuries usually result from gunshot or shrapnel wounds but may also occur in traffic and industrial accidents or from assaults with blunt weapons. A neurosurgeon must treat such injuries immediately by cleansing the wound, removing foreign matter, and repairing tissue.

CLOSED HEAD INJURIES

Closed head injuries, which do not penetrate the scalp and skull, are much more common than penetrating injuries. The person's level of consciousness after the injury is the best indicator of whether the effects will be mild or severe. In 20 to 30 percent of fatal head injuries, the skull

HOW DOES DAMAGE OCCUR IN A CLOSED HEAD INJURY?

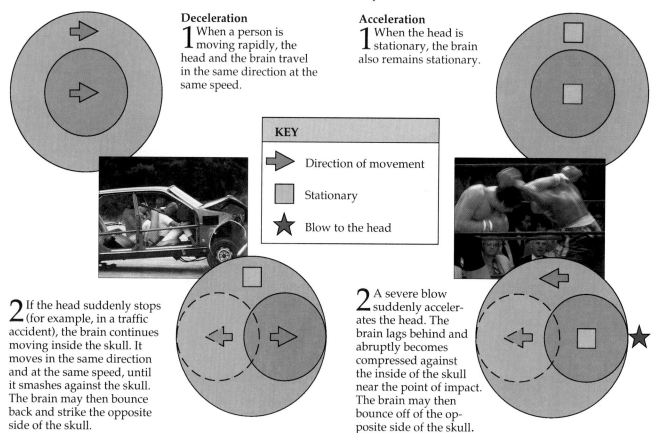

Deceleration
1 When a person is moving rapidly, the head and the brain travel in the same direction at the same speed.

Acceleration
1 When the head is stationary, the brain also remains stationary.

KEY

- Direction of movement
- Stationary
- Blow to the head

2 If the head suddenly stops (for example, in a traffic accident), the brain continues moving inside the skull. It moves in the same direction and at the same speed, until it smashes against the skull. The brain may then bounce back and strike the opposite side of the skull.

2 A severe blow suddenly accelerates the head. The brain lags behind and abruptly becomes compressed against the inside of the skull near the point of impact. The brain may then bounce off of the opposite side of the skull.

Bleeding inside the skull

Torn blood vessels cause bleeding inside the skull. Bleeding may take place after minor injuries, especially in older people. Bleeding may occur between the dura mater and the arachnoid (subdural hemorrhage) or, less commonly, between the inner surface of the skull and the dura mater (epidural hemorrhage).

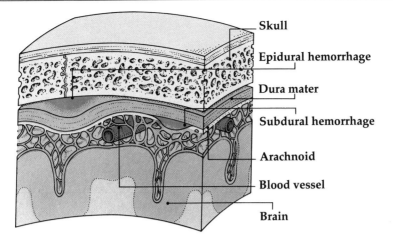

- Skull
- Epidural hemorrhage
- Dura mater
- Subdural hemorrhage
- Arachnoid
- Blood vessel
- Brain

WHAT IS A CONCUSSION?

Concussion is a state of immediate but temporary loss of brain function without obvious signs of physical damage to the brain. The period of unconsciousness may last for seconds, minutes, or hours, but complete recovery occurs within 24 hours. Concussion follows sudden acceleration or deceleration of the brain that can cause rotational motion or sliding, but the exact cause of the loss of function remains uncertain. It is not due to temporary loss of blood supply, as in a TIA (see page 109).

remains intact. This is why doctors use computed tomography (CT) scanning to detect internal bleeding or other abnormalities.

In a closed head injury, damage to the brain most often follows sudden deceleration or acceleration of the head (see page 122). The brain simply may not function normally for a few minutes to a few hours, even though no structural damage has been done. This condition is called a concussion and usually includes a brief loss of consciousness. More severe injuries may cut the brain or severely bruise it as a result of impact against the inside of the skull. Injuries may also displace or crush the brain into open spaces in the skull, such as the opening at its base for the spinal cord. Blood vessels may tear as a result of rotational forces or skull fracture.

person's symptoms. Bleeding inside the skull (see above) may not cause immediate symptoms. For an hour or two ("the lucid interval"), the victim may appear normal. In some cases, bleeding is slow and intermittent, and symptoms may not occur for days, weeks, or months. Later symptoms may include headache, confusion, drowsiness, apathy, change in personality or behavior, and sometimes a seizure. Such symptoms require immediate hospital treatment.

SYMPTOMS AND SIGNS

Most people who receive head injuries are briefly stunned but do not lose consciousness. Often their only symptom is a minor headache. More severe head injuries may bring about a period of unconsciousness or even coma. People who lose consciousness experience brief memory loss for the event and sometimes for a period before and after the event. Paralysis, loss of sensation, and muscular weakness head the list of other severe head injury symptoms. The area of brain tissue injured determines the

HELPLINE
SUDDEN UNEXPLAINED DROWSINESS

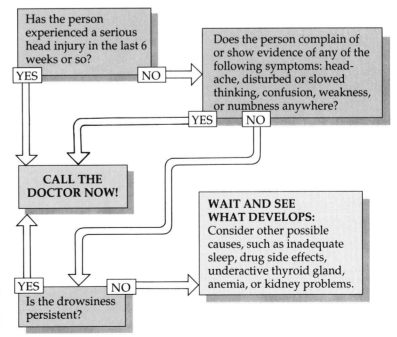

Has the person experienced a serious head injury in the last 6 weeks or so? YES NO

Does the person complain of or show evidence of any of the following symptoms: headache, disturbed or slowed thinking, confusion, weakness, or numbness anywhere? YES NO

CALL THE DOCTOR NOW!

WAIT AND SEE WHAT DEVELOPS: Consider other possible causes, such as inadequate sleep, drug side effects, underactive thyroid gland, anemia, or kidney problems.

YES NO

Is the drowsiness persistent?

NECK INJURY

Serious neck injuries can severely damage the spinal cord. Usually protected by the spinal column, the spinal cord can be crushed or severed when vertebral bones are displaced. The spinal cord can also be injured when cancerous vertebrae collapse.

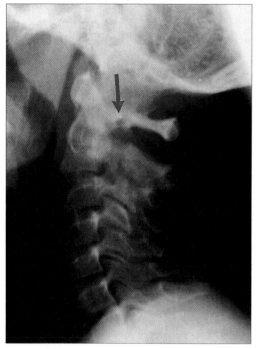

Neck fracture
This side-view X-ray shows a fracture of the second cervical vertebra (arrow). Such a fracture may be caused by falling or by slipping under a seat belt.

Compression of the spinal cord occurs when a protruding disc or tumor presses on the spinal canal. Damage to the spinal cord at neck level causes loss of movement, sensation, and autonomic nervous system function below the level of injury (see PARALYSIS on page 126). The higher up the spinal cord the damage occurs, the more serious the effects.

Spinal cord injuries usually happen when the spine is both fractured and dislocated. Such serious injuries usually result from falls, knife wounds, accidents from diving into shallow water, motor-vehicle accidents, industrial accidents, and gunshot wounds. Whiplash injuries can also damage the spinal cord.

POSTTRAUMATIC SYNDROME

Following severe head injuries, many people develop a disorder known as posttraumatic syndrome. People injured in frightening circumstances, such as an assault, a plane crash, or a war, are more likely to develop the syndrome than are those injured in an accident at home. Symptoms include headache, anxiety, and loss of energy. In more severe cases, personality and behavioral abnormalities occur. The most severe cases are characterized by loss of intellectual capacity, judgment, and memory. In most affected people, posttraumatic syndrome tends to abate in several weeks or months.

Treatment of neck injury

The victim of a possible neck injury should be moved only by people trained in emergency medical care. Doctors will obtain X-rays of the spine to confirm the diagnosis made after taking the person's medical history and giving him or her a physical examination. To assess the extent of damage, doctors may also obtain an MRI or CT scan.

Treatment usually involves surgical or nonsurgical realignment of the spine and also head traction to hold the bones in position until healing takes place. To apply head traction, doctors lie the victim flat and fasten weighted metal tongs onto the skull.

Effects of a neck injury

The outcome of a neck injury depends primarily on its severity and location. About 10 percent of people with broken necks die of the injury. Some must be kept alive on a respirator because their breathing muscles are paralyzed. Others become quadriplegic (paralyzed from the neck downward). A realignment of the neck bones can prevent permanent injury to the spinal cord.

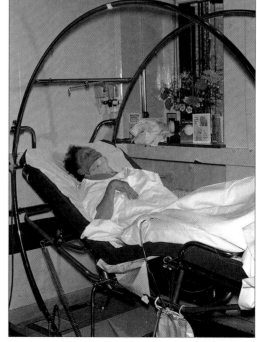

Stryker frame
Doctors usually treat a patient with a spinal cord injury on a special bed called a Stryker frame. The bed allows the person to be turned with minimal disturbance of his or her position.

CASE HISTORY
A BUMP ON THE HEAD

Burt is a lively **youngster. One day he fell off his bicycle, badly bumping and bruising his forehead. Burt seemed fine at first but was unusually quiet that afternoon. Later, Burt's mother found him lying on his bed. He complained of a headache and seemed confused and drowsy. His parents called their doctor, who told them to take Burt to the hospital if he became more drowsy. He did and they rushed Burt to the emergency room.**

PERSONAL DETAILS
Name Burt Macleod
Age 10
Occupation Student
Family Burt has three older sisters. His parents and sisters are all in good health.

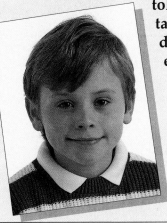

MEDICAL BACKGROUND
Although somewhat accident-prone, Burt has always been healthy.

THE CONSULTATION
By the time Burt arrives at the emergency room, he is in a deep coma. The doctors recognize that severe pressure has developed in Burt's skull. They give Burt mannitol, a drug that temporarily decreases the pressure in his skull, and put him on a respirator, a machine that helps him breathe.

FURTHER INVESTIGATION
An immediate computed tomography (CT) scan shows an extensive blood clot in the epidural space pressing on Burt's brain and a fracture of the left temporal bone of Burt's skull.

THE DIAGNOSIS
The neurosurgeon shows Burt's mother and father the scan and explains that Burt has suffered an EPIDURAL HEMORRHAGE, resulting from bleeding of the middle meningeal artery, which was torn by the skull fracture. An expanding blood clot is compressing Burt's brain, placing him in serious danger. The surgeon explains that progressive brain compression invariably leads to deepening coma and eventually death. Only immediate surgery can save Burt's life. Burt's parents agree to surgery and sign a consent form. Burt is immediately taken to the operating room where he undergoes an operation to remove the blood clot.

THE TREATMENT
After making a skin incision, the neurosurgeon drills a hole in Burt's skull and allows the blood clot to drain. The neurosurgeon then identifies the bleeding artery and ties it off. The neurosurgeon checks other surrounding structures for damage but finds none. Before closing the incision, the neurosurgeon makes certain the bleeding has stopped.

THE FOLLOW-UP
Burt makes a rapid and uncomplicated recovery from surgery. He experiences no further symptoms of drowsiness or other complications from the fall he suffered. When he returns to school, he finds his classmates are fascinated by his shaven head and the scar on his scalp. His parents are tempted to try to limit Burt's activities, but the doctor warns them not to become overprotective toward their son.

The operation
After removing the blood clot, the neurosurgeon is able to see bleeding from the middle meningeal artery. He secures the artery with forceps and ties it off tightly.

Ties   Forceps

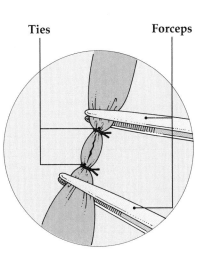

Site of bleeding
Middle meningeal artery

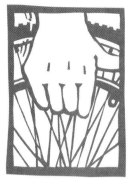

PARALYSIS

WE TAKE ease of movement for granted. Walking through the woods, stretching after a good night's sleep, or reaching up to a shelf, we move our limbs without a second thought. For a person whose limbs are paralyzed, life is drastically altered by the inability to perform these movements. Damage to any part of the motor system – the motor areas of the brain, the nerve tracts that extend down the spinal cord, the nerves that supply the muscles, or the muscles themselves – can cause paralysis.

The extent of paralysis depends on which part of the motor system is damaged. Sometimes people experience loss of sensation and movement in the paralyzed body part. Paralyzed muscles are either more stiff or more floppy than normal. Chances for recovery tend to be better when damage affects the peripheral rather than the central nervous system.

WHAT CAUSES PARALYSIS?

Motor system functions can be affected by such factors as physical damage, infection, poisoning by a toxin or metal, disturbance of blood supply, tumor, nutritional deficiency, or developmental abnormality. Damage to the insulating

TYPES OF PARALYSIS

Types of paralysis differ depending on the extent of damage a person's motor system has sustained, as illustrated here. Damage to motor areas on one side of the brain causes paralysis of the opposite side of the person's body. Complete destruction of the spinal cord results in total paralysis and loss of sensation below the level of injury. Neck injury causes paralysis of the trunk and all four limbs. If the damage is below a certain level in the neck, the victim will still be able to breathe on his or her own. An injury high in the neck or in the lower part of the brain is often fatal. Those who survive suffer paralysis of all four limbs, the trunk, and the respiratory (breathing) muscles. People with such an injury can live only with the help of a respirator. An injury to the spinal cord below the level of the neck does not affect the arms but paralyzes the trunk and legs.

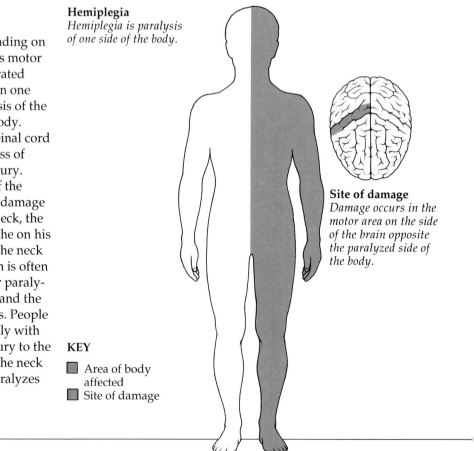

Hemiplegia
Hemiplegia is paralysis of one side of the body.

Site of damage
Damage occurs in the motor area on the side of the brain opposite the paralyzed side of the body.

KEY
- Area of body affected
- Site of damage

myelin sheaths of the nerve fibers, as occurs in cases of multiple sclerosis, can also cause paralysis (see page 130).

The most common cause of hemiplegia (paralysis of one side of the body) is stroke (see page 106). Hemiplegia may also result from such disorders as a brain abscess or tumor, head trauma, or a severe infection that causes inflammation of the brain (encephalitis).

Injury to the spinal cord, often a result of a motor-vehicle accident, is the most common cause of paraplegia (paralysis of both legs) and quadriplegia (paralysis of the trunk and all four limbs). This type of injury may also cause loss of sensation and loss of bladder and bowel control. Other causes of paraplegia include accidents from diving into shallow water, multiple sclerosis, tumors, progressive narrowing of the spinal canal, or severe infection of the spinal cord.

COPING WITH A SEVERE SPINAL INJURY

With the use of mobility aids, such as wheelchairs and specially designed automobiles, paraplegics can lead relatively independent lives. Sexual function often remains viable. But quadriplegics must rely on others to assist with activities of daily living such as eating and bathing.

Mobility

Many paraplegics acquire a remarkable degree of wheelchair mobility. In addition, wheelchair ramps and wide doorways allow greater access to public facilities. Homes and cars can also be modified to allow greater freedom of movement. Many communities offer van services to the disabled, either free or at a minimal cost.

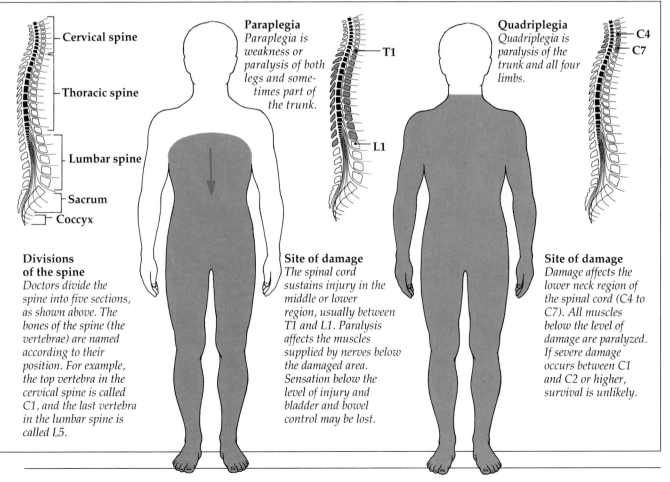

Cervical spine

Thoracic spine

Lumbar spine

Sacrum

Coccyx

Divisions of the spine
Doctors divide the spine into five sections, as shown above. The bones of the spine (the vertebrae) are named according to their position. For example, the top vertebra in the cervical spine is called C1, and the last vertebra in the lumbar spine is called L5.

Paraplegia
Paraplegia is weakness or paralysis of both legs and sometimes part of the trunk.

T1

L1

Site of damage
The spinal cord sustains injury in the middle or lower region, usually between T1 and L1. Paralysis affects the muscles supplied by nerves below the damaged area. Sensation below the level of injury and bladder and bowel control may be lost.

Quadriplegia
Quadriplegia is paralysis of the trunk and all four limbs.

C4

C7

Site of damage
Damage affects the lower neck region of the spinal cord (C4 to C7). All muscles below the level of damage are paralyzed. If severe damage occurs between C1 and C2 or higher, survival is unlikely.

Special problems after spinal injury

People with limited mobility must avoid sitting or lying in one position for a long period. Bed sores can develop, particularly over bony parts of the body. Paraplegics and quadriplegics must also

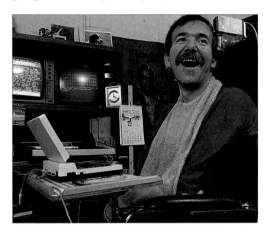

Working from home
There is increasing potential for disabled people to work at home, linked to a business center by modem, facsimile, and computer networks. Technological developments have also enabled quadriplegics to operate computers via special headsets that interpret head or mouth movements.

cope with loss of bladder control. A tube (catheter) inserted into the bladder allows urine to drain into a plastic bag. But even with careful attention, prolonged use of catheters often leads to infection of the bladder and even the kidneys. Some

SUPPORT GROUPS

The following national organizations offer counseling and advice to paraplegics and quadriplegics:
◆ National Spinal Cord Injury Association, 600 W. Cummings Park, Woburn, MA 01801 (800-962-9629)
◆ National Rehabilitation Information Center, 8455 Colesville Rd., Suite 935, Silver Spring, MD 20910 (800-346-2742)
◆ Mobility International USA, P.O. Box 3551, Eugene, OR 97403 (503-343-1284)
◆ National Information Center for Handicapped Children and Youth, P.O. Box 1492, Washington, DC 20013 (703-893-6061)
◆ National Wheelchair Athletic Association, 3595 E.Fountain Blvd., Suite L1, Colorado Springs, CO 80910 (719-574-1150)

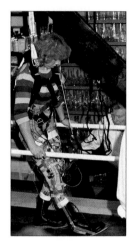

Helpful technology
Bioengineering research is attempting to develop devices that provide computer-controlled muscle stimulation so that paraplegics can stand and even walk. The technology is still at an early stage, but progress is being made.

paraplegics who have lost control of bladder function can learn to empty the bladder at intervals by pressing on the lower abdomen.

Psychological adjustment

Many people who suffer severe spinal injury are young and otherwise healthy. The resentment and bitterness they feel because of their disability are understandable. These people need strong positive motivation to deal with the major psychological adjustment demanded by disability. Many rehabilitation facilities do well in generating a positive attitude in their patients. But the support of family, friends, and health professionals can contribute greatly to the disabled person's quality of life.

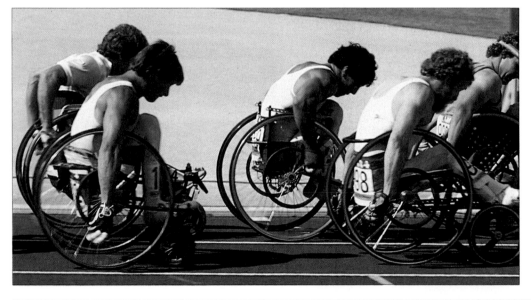

Recreation
Many paraplegics participate in athletic competitions. Some take part in long-distance races, such as marathons, at local and international levels.

CEREBRAL PALSY

Cerebral palsy affects about one in 500 children. Some affected children show only the slightest disability, while others are almost totally disabled. Cerebral palsy results from damage to motor parts of the brain during fetal or early childhood development.

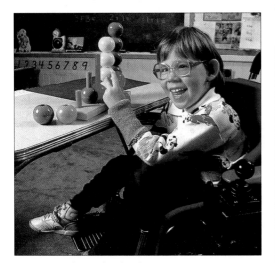

Living with cerebral palsy
Parents of a child with cerebral palsy have a demanding role, but careful medical management, including physical therapy, can do much to help the child. Surgery can sometimes improve function. Mildly affected children can usually attend schools with normal children. The more severely affected require special schools.

Experts once believed that injury and lack of oxygen at the time of birth caused cerebral palsy. They now recognize that brain damage often occurs before birth, but the reasons remain unclear. Meningitis, encephalitis, head injury early in life, and many other conditions can also lead to cerebral palsy.

Effects of cerebral palsy

Children who have cerebral palsy display abnormal movement with muscle stiffness (spastic paralysis). Difficulty in walking varies. Children often have a "scissors gait," in which the legs press tightly together and rub against each other. Paralysis is often limited to the legs, but may involve the arms as well.

Cerebral palsy may not be recognized until well into the baby's first year. About half of children with cerebral palsy are mentally retarded, with an IQ below 70. A parallel relationship usually exists between the extent of paralysis and the severity of the mental defect.

Speech articulation may be affected. About one fourth of children who have cerebral palsy experience seizures. The disease is incurable but physical and speech therapies can improve function.

FACIAL PALSY

Facial palsy, also known as Bell's palsy, is a fairly common disorder in which the muscles of expression on one side of the face become paralyzed due to damage to the facial nerve that supplies them. The facial paralysis may be total or partial, depending on the severity of nerve damage. Partial paralysis is reversible and usually resolves in several weeks or months. Some people with total paralysis recover fully, but many experience severe disfigurement. Plastic surgery is an option in such cases.

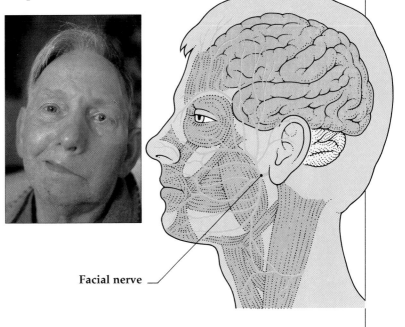

Facial nerve

How does facial palsy occur?
On each side of the face, the facial nerve passes through a narrow channel in the temporal bone. Inflammation from a viral infection or some other cause leads to swelling and compression of the nerve so that it cannot conduct impulses to the muscles. Within a few hours of onset, the affected side of the face becomes flattened and expressionless. The corner of the mouth and the lower eyelid sag downward (above left) and the person cannot close the upper eyelid.

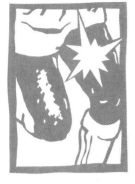

MULTIPLE SCLEROSIS

MULTIPLE SCLEROSIS is a progressive central nervous system disease that follows a breakdown of the myelin sheaths that protect and insulate nerve fibers. Symptoms vary among affected people, and disease progression can follow different patterns. The onset of multiple sclerosis usually occurs in the early to middle 20s but can begin at any age between 12 and 50.

Multiple sclerosis occurs more commonly in women than in men. The annual incidence of the disease in the US is roughly two in every 100,000 people.

Medical science has yet to discover the cause of multiple sclerosis. The disease seems to occur more commonly in temperate climates than in tropical areas. Recent studies show a relationship between the risk of developing multiple sclerosis and the region in which victims lived during their first 15 years. This finding has led many medical experts to believe that the disease may originate from early exposure to a virus that remains latent in the brain and/or spinal cord and becomes active later in life. The disease also has a genetic component.

WHAT ARE THE SYMPTOMS?

The most common initial symptom of multiple sclerosis is numbness or tingling in the hands or feet. Less often, sufferers notice visual disturbances,

PREVALENCE OF MULTIPLE SCLEROSIS

The occurrence of multiple sclerosis varies widely among different regions and ethnic groups. The highest known prevalence worldwide is in the Orkney islands in Great Britain, where as many as three in 1,000 people have the disease. In contrast, multiple sclerosis is almost nonexistent among black African groups and Eskimos living in their native countries. It is the most common acquired nervous system disease in young adults.

WHAT IS MULTIPLE SCLEROSIS?

The fatty myelin sheaths that surround nerve fibers are essential for normal transmission of nerve impulses to and from the brain. In multiple sclerosis, the myelin sheaths of some nerve fibers break down, interrupting impulse transmission.

If a significant number of nerve fibers are demyelinated, the affected part of the central nervous system develops a damaged area called a plaque. The exact sites of the plaques determine the symptoms the person will experience.

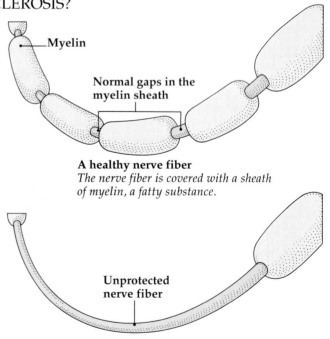

A healthy nerve fiber
The nerve fiber is covered with a sheath of myelin, a fatty substance.

A demyelinated nerve fiber
The myelin sheath has degenerated, leaving an unprotected area of nerve fiber that prevents transmission of signals to and from the brain.

muscle weakness, slow movement, balance problems or dizziness, bladder problems, or loss of sensation in the face as first signs of the disease. These symptoms often disappear after a few weeks, a process called remission. After months or years, symptoms may return, a process called relapse.

Multiple sclerosis is progressive, meaning symptoms gradually get worse. People with the disease may find it increasingly difficult to maintain their independence because of muscle weakness or stiffness, loss of sensation in the hands and feet, pain, fatigue, incontinence, and personality changes.

DIAGNOSIS

When diagnosing multiple sclerosis, doctors usually try to rule out other disorders. Magnetic resonance imaging (MRI) can be used to identify multiple sclerosis lesions (plaques).

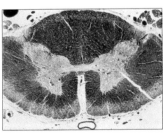

Normal spinal cord

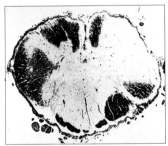

Spinal cord of a person with multiple sclerosis

Plaques inside the spinal column
Damage from multiple sclerosis is apparent in the comparison of two cross-sections through the spinal cord shown above. The upper cross-section shows a healthy spinal cord, where the nerve fibers can transmit impulses to and from the brain. The lower cross-section shows a spinal cord with damaged areas, or plaques, that block transmission.

THE EFFECTS OF MULTIPLE SCLEROSIS

Because different parts of the central nervous system control specific bodily functions, the symptoms of multiple sclerosis manifest in many different ways. The symptoms may vary in location, type, and severity, and one person may experience varying symptoms at different stages of the disease.

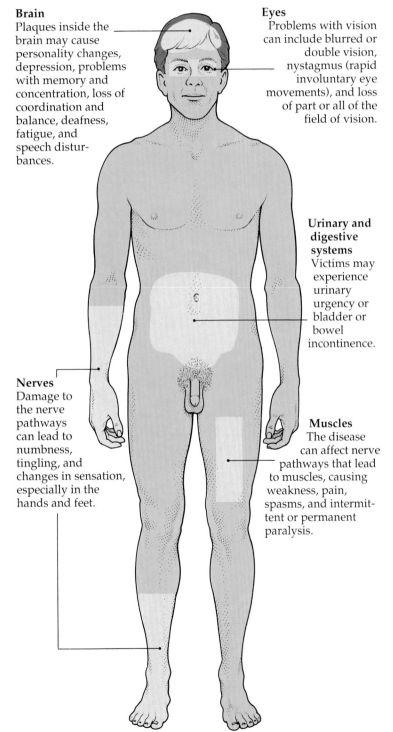

Brain
Plaques inside the brain may cause personality changes, depression, problems with memory and concentration, loss of coordination and balance, deafness, fatigue, and speech disturbances.

Eyes
Problems with vision can include blurred or double vision, nystagmus (rapid involuntary eye movements), and loss of part or all of the field of vision.

Urinary and digestive systems
Victims may experience urinary urgency or bladder or bowel incontinence.

Nerves
Damage to the nerve pathways can lead to numbness, tingling, and changes in sensation, especially in the hands and feet.

Muscles
The disease can affect nerve pathways that lead to muscles, causing weakness, pain, spasms, and intermittent or permanent paralysis.

HOW THE DISEASE PROGRESSES

The progression of multiple sclerosis can follow several different patterns. Some people experience a severe initial attack followed by a remission of symptoms for several decades. Others suffer slow degeneration relieved by periods of remission, while a small percentage of people undergo a rapid, unrelieved degeneration.

Disability level

Time

LIVING WITH MULTIPLE SCLEROSIS

Whatever pattern of multiple sclerosis you have, you can adapt your life-style in various ways to maximize the mobility that you still retain.

◆ Keep your weight down
◆ Avoid alcohol and don't smoke
◆ Eat a healthy, balanced diet
◆ Exercise regularly (swimming is particularly good)
◆ Get enough sleep and rest
◆ Avoid hot atmospheres and climates
◆ Join a multiple sclerosis self-help group

TREATMENT

There is no cure for multiple sclerosis. Treatment focuses on relief of symptoms. Because doctors believe that myelin breakdown occurs when the immune system attacks the nerve fibers, the most promising area of treatment involves an alteration of the immune response. Acute relapses generally respond to treatment with adrenocorticotropic hormone (ACTH) or prednisone, a corticosteroid drug. Researchers are also investigating newer treatments with stronger immunosuppressant drugs. These treatments can temporarily relieve symptoms in many victims but have no long-term effect on the course of the disease.

Unusual therapies, such as treatment with oxygen in a pressure chamber and injections of snake venom, have been used in attempts to relieve symptoms. These have not proved beneficial. Some sufferers believe that a diet free of gluten (grain protein) or one that includes a high intake of polyunsaturated oils relieves their symptoms, but the effectiveness of these diets has not been proven.

Physical and occupational therapies can improve functional ability. A positive mental attitude helps the person cope with the effects of progressive physical limitations.

OUTLOOK

The multiple sclerosis relapse rate tends to be highest in the first few years of the disease. Prospects for remaining symptom-free improve the longer a person remains free from an attack. After 25 years, of those persons still alive, one third still work, one third have altered their life-style but are independent, and one third require help with activities of daily living. The later in life that multiple sclerosis first appears, the more likely the symptoms are to be chronic (continuous) and progressive.

CASE HISTORY
SUDDEN BLURRED VISION

ONE MORNING AT WORK, **Susan experienced a sudden blurring of her vision while reading a memo. Blinking did not clear her vision. When she closed her left eye, the words directly in front of her seemed to disappear. She also noticed that she could not see colors properly with her right eye. Alarmed, she immediately called her doctor.**

PERSONAL DETAILS
Name Susan Taylor
Age 36
Occupation Personnel assistant
Family Susan is divorced with no children. Her parents are both healthy. Susan's grandmother had multiple sclerosis.

MEDICAL BACKGROUND
Susan is generally healthy but recently had the flu, from which she recovered without complications.

THE CONSULTATION
Susan's doctor performs a full physical examination. When he examines her eyes, he finds that both her retinas and optic discs, the part of the optic nerve inside the eye, look normal. He refers Susan to a neuro-ophthalmologist for further tests.

THE SPECIALIST CONSULTATION
The neuro-ophthalmologist tests Susan's visual field (the area she can see to each side without moving her head) and finds that she is blind in the center of the right visual field (a condition called central scotoma). Testing shows that she has lost color vision in her right eye. Vision in the left eye is normal. The specialist finds no evidence of any other neurological disease but, to be on the safe side, arranges for her to have a computed tomography (CT) scan.

THE DIAGNOSIS
The CT scan shows no visible abnormality in Susan's brain and no evidence of any pressure on the optic nerve. The specialist tells Susan that a central scotoma and loss of color vision are usually signs of OPTIC NEURITIS. This type of inflammation of the optic nerve is often caused by multiple sclerosis (a progressive disease of the central nervous system with a wide range of symptoms). She explains that when optic neuritis is the only neurological abnormality present, no reliable diagnostic tests can confirm whether the underlying cause is multiple sclerosis. But she tells Susan that optic neuritis should be regarded as a warning sign, especially because her grandmother had multiple sclerosis.

The specialist explains that in cases of multiple sclerosis, the first (and sometimes the only) manifestation of the disease occurs after an illness, such as her recent case of the flu. The specialist informs her that many people with optic neuritis do not develop other signs of multiple sclerosis and that optic neuritis clears up completely in one third of people.

THE TREATMENT
Because the only treatment recommended for her condition is rest, Susan arranges to take some time off from work.

THE OUTCOME
Susan's vision returns to normal within a few weeks. She decides to think positively, to live life to the fullest, and to stay as healthy as possible. In this way, she will be in the best position to deal with multiple sclerosis should further symptoms develop.

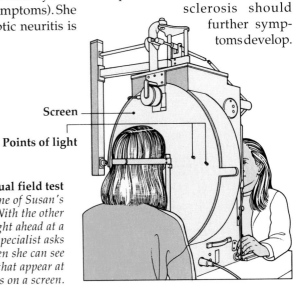

Screen

Points of light

Visual field test
During the test, one of Susan's eyes is covered. With the other eye, she looks straight ahead at a fixed point. The specialist asks her to say when she can see points of light that appear at different places on a screen.

DEMENTIA

I MAGINE BEING able to remember the day you were married but not being able to recall what season it is or the name of the town in which you now live. In cases of dementia, intellect and memory decline and personality deteriorates. This frightening condition causes a group of symptoms to appear that get progressively worse.

While mild memory impairment can occur with aging, dementia is not the usual consequence of old age. But the risk of dementia does increase with age. The previous distinction between senile dementia, occurring in the elderly, and presenile dementia no longer applies because doctors now realize that the disease is the same at any age.

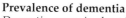

Prevalence of dementia
Dementia occurs in about 2 percent of people between the ages of 65 and 75 and in up to 15 percent of people older than 80. With increased life expectancy in the US (more than 75 percent of people can expect to reach age 60), the number of elderly people will increase by 20 percent by the year 2000. The number of people with dementia will correspondingly escalate. The predicted number of people who will have dementia in the US during the next half century is shown in this graph.

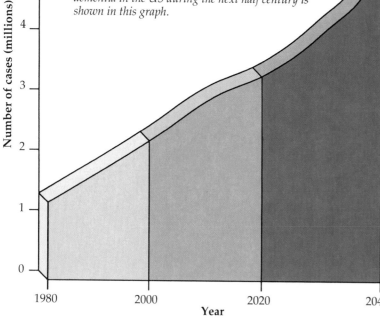

Number of cases (millions)

Year

CAUSES OF DEMENTIA

Dementia can arise from a number of different causes, the most common of which are described below.

Alzheimer's disease

Alzheimer's disease accounts for about 55 percent of all cases of dementia. But doctors usually make only a presumptive diagnosis following a physical and psychological examination of a person suspected of having Alzheimer's disease. The only way doctors can diagnose the disease with certainty is by examining brain tissue after the person has died.

A person with Alzheimer's disease shows a gradual, progressive decline in mental functions. The cause or causes of the disease have yet to be identified, but doctors suspect one possibility is an environmental factor. Studies show that patients with the disease have low levels of the neurotransmitter acetylcholine in

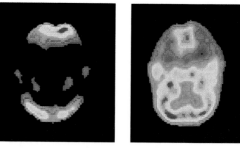

Decreased brain activity in Alzheimer's disease
A positron emission tomography (PET) scan of the brain of someone with Alzheimer's disease (above left) shows lower metabolic activity compared with a healthy person's brain (above right). The brightest areas show the highest metabolic activity.

their brains. This chemical is crucial for learning and memory functions. Some of the changes that occur in the brains of people with Alzheimer's disease are shown in the photo at right.

Multi-infarct dementia

Multi-infarct dementia is responsible for 15 percent of dementia cases and arises from the destruction of brain tissue following multiple tiny strokes. A person with this form of dementia may have a history of other illnesses that require treatment, such as stroke, diabetes, hypertension, or cardiovascular disease. Multi-infarct dementia can appear quickly. Deterioration occurs in "steps."

Dementia caused by infections

Creutzfeldt-Jakob disease is a form of dementia thought to be caused by a slow virus – one that remains in nerve cells a long time before showing its effects. People with Creutzfeldt-Jakob disease display the symptoms of dementia along with involuntary jerking movements. Dementia related to acquired immune deficiency syndrome (AIDS) is now a common form of dementia caused by infection. Many people with AIDS develop dementia. People who care for those with forms of dementia caused by infection should consult their doctor about the need to protect themselves from contact with the person's bodily

How Alzheimer's disease changes the brain
Changes seen in the brains of people with Alzheimer's disease include neuritic plaques (arrow), which contain abnormal deposits of a protein, and neurofibrillary tangles (abnormal fiberlike tangles of protein inside nerve cells).

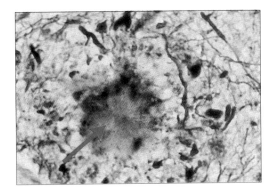

fluids. For example, they may be told to wear disposable plastic or rubber gloves when cleaning up bodily fluids or when changing bedding.

SYMPTOMS OF DEMENTIA

The symptoms, diagnostic methods, and management problems are similar for all irreversible forms of dementia. But because Alzheimer's disease is the most common form of dementia, its symptoms deserve a thorough description.

Early in the course of the disease, the person with Alzheimer's disease has periods of forgetfulness. He or she may be unable to remember a doctor's appointment or may not know what day it is. These first signs are difficult to distinguish from the normal forgetfulness that occurs in old age or with bereavement and other forms of severe stress.

In the later stages of the disease, personality changes become apparent, such

ALCOHOL-RELATED DEMENTIAS

Excess alcohol intake can cause a variety of dementias. Heavy alcohol consumption kills nerve cells and causes the brain to shrink. In addition, liver failure from chronic alcoholism can further impair mental ability. The chronic alcoholic also frequently neglects his or her diet, becoming deficient in thiamine (vitamin B_1). This deficiency leads to Wernicke's encephalopathy, a reversible syndrome marked by confusion, unsteady gait, and abnormal eye movements. If alcohol consumption continues and the thiamine deficiency is not corrected, mental functions may become permanently impaired.

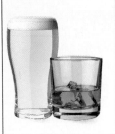

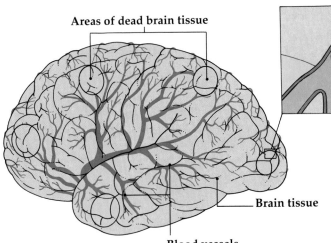

Areas of dead brain tissue

Brain tissue

Blood vessels

Blocked blood vessel

Strokes throughout the brain
In multi-infarct dementia, the effects of many small or large strokes accumulate, causing progressive damage to widespread areas of brain tissue where blood vessels have become blocked. Preventive measures, such as controlling blood cholesterol levels and blood pressure, can help prevent or delay further strokes or a series of strokes.

Problems of Alzheimer's disease
As the disease progresses, the person experiences periods of confusion. He or she may find simple tasks difficult, such as telling time or tying a shoelace. The person may become lost in a previously familiar environment and may be unable to grasp what is going on around him or her.

as sudden, unpredictable mood changes, anxiety and agitation, distress, or embarrassing behavior. The person increasingly neglects personal hygiene, loses bladder control, and cannot take care of the routine activities of daily life. Speech often becomes incoherent. The sufferer becomes increasingly unaware of his or her condition and is not able to recognize even close family members, friends, or his or her spouse.

DIAGNOSIS

Many older people who experience confusion and poor memory do not have Alzheimer's disease or another type of irreversible dementia. Doctors must rule out all disorders that can cause similar symptoms before making a diagnosis of dementia. To accomplish this, doctors perform a physical examination and order neuropsychological tests.

Physical examination
The doctor performs a physical examination and a series of tests designed primarily to exclude treatable causes of dementia, such as heart, liver, or kidney failure; thyroid dysfunction (especially underactivity); vitamin B_{12} deficiency; and hypoglycemia (low blood sugar level). Rarer neurological disorders, such

The behavior profile
If you are the caregiver to a person suspected of having Alzheimer's disease, you may find it useful to keep a record of difficulties the person experiences, such as behavior problems and memory loss. This record can help the doctor make an accurate diagnosis.

as syphilis of the brain, must also be ruled out. Brain imaging techniques, such as computed tomography (CT) scanning or magnetic resonance imaging (MRI), may exclude other causes of symptoms, such as a tumor or a stroke.

Neuropsychological tests
The doctor then performs tests of mental status and functioning. A person who has dementia will show clear evidence of defects in judgment and awareness, such as failure to remember a simple set of numbers or an address. Psychological tests can help confirm a suspected diagnosis of dementia, determine how far the disease has progressed, and help eliminate the possibility of depression, which may mimic dementia in the elderly.

TREATMENT

No cure exists for progressive forms of dementia such as Alzheimer's disease. Treatment prescribed by a doctor emphasizes relieving symptoms and keeping the person comfortable. Good personal care, clean and comfortable surroundings, and a nutritious diet form the basics of custodial care. Sedatives can help reduce restlessness or agitation but sometimes have the opposite effect.

CASE HISTORY
MENTAL DETERIORATION

DURING THE YEARS **that she lived with her daughter Vera, Elsie had gradually become confused about where she was living and who Vera was. One day, Elsie turned on the gas stove and let the flame burn for no reason. Another day, she wandered away from the house and got lost. When Elsie became unable to control her bladder, Vera called a gerontologist.**

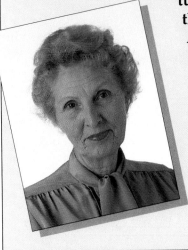

PERSONAL DETAILS
Name Elsie Polcic
Age 73
Occupation Retired
Family Mother died at age 75; father was killed in World War I.

MEDICAL BACKGROUND
Elsie has never smoked cigarettes or drunk alcohol. She has suffered from respiratory disease since she was a child and now has chronic bronchitis, for which she sometimes needs antibiotics. But she has always been active and, until 3 years ago, took a long walk every day.

THE CONSULTATION
The gerontologist gives Elsie a full physical examination and, apart from the bronchitis, finds few physical explanations for her recent deterioration. He decides to perform some cognitive (mental judgment and awareness) tests. A doctor uses these tests when he or she suspects that a person has suffered the type of mental deterioration caused by dementia, brain tumor, depression, or stroke. The doctor asks Elsie to perform simple mental exercises, such as subtracting one number from another, and to answer basic questions about current affairs, such as the name of the President. He also asks Elsie to tell him the day, month, and year. Elsie fails all these tests. The gerontologist, suspecting some form of dementia, arranges for CT scanning and additional blood tests.

THE INVESTIGATIONS AND DIAGNOSIS
Results of all blood tests are normal. The CT scan shows no evidence of stroke or brain damage. But the fluid-filled ventricles of Elsie's brain are enlarged, and her brain has obviously shrunk. These are characteristics often seen on the CT scans of people with ALZHEIMER'S DISEASE. Unfortunately, no other safe and simple tests are available to confirm the diagnosis. In the absence of any other cause, the gerontologist tells Vera that the diagnosis of Alzheimer's disease is most likely.

THE SPECIALIST'S ADVICE
The gerontologist explains to Vera that there is no treatment for Alzheimer's disease. He tells Vera that, since the disease is progressive, Elsie's forgetfulness will continue to increase. The gerontologist knows that Vera has been finding it increasingly difficult to cope with Elsie's constant need for care. The doctor tells Vera that she should not feel guilty about relinquishing her caregiver's role. Vera visits a nursing home just down the street that a social worker has recommended. She is impressed with the facilities and pleasant atmosphere and feels reassured by the staff's caring attitude. The cost of care is high, but Elsie's savings and assets should cover most of the cost for some time.

THE OUTCOME
Vera decides to place Elsie in the care of the nursing home. This move frees Vera from worry about her mother's safety and the demands of constant care. She now has the opportunity to reestablish a close, loving relationship with her mother, knowing that Elsie is being well cared for.

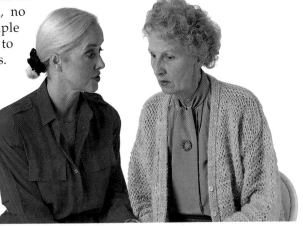

Happily settled
Elsie quickly adjusts to life in the nursing home and seems comfortable there. Vera visits her every day.

LIVING WITH DEMENTIA

The vast majority of people who have dementia remain in the familiar surroundings of home, in the care of a family member. The caregiver is usually extremely reluctant to send the dementia sufferer to a nursing home, and in-home nursing care costs can be prohibitive. Coming to terms with dementia in a family member means accepting loss and coping with bereavement for the person long before he or she dies. An affected spouse or parent may no longer have the personality, special qualities, and competencies of the person the caregiver once knew so well. Despite this loss, the caregiver must show patience, understanding, and kindness while on many occasions feeling anger, resentment, frustration, and guilt. Such mixed emotions are natural and normal.

If you are caring for a person with dementia, you can take a number of steps to make things a little easier.

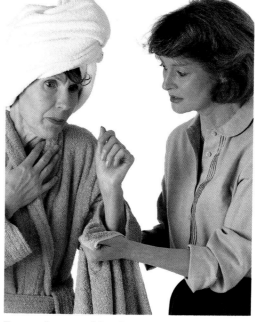

Personal care and hygiene
A person with dementia may forget whether he or she has bathed or shaved and may need a reminder. Allow the person to perform as much of a task as possible. You may need to supervise shaving or bathing for safety purposes, but try to make these occasions pleasant.

WANDERING

The confused dementia sufferer often wanders aimlessly. When this happens, try to distract and coax the person rather than confronting him or her. Install locks that are difficult to operate, and place them at the bottom of the doors. Have the person wear an identification bracelet that lists his or her name, address, and telephone number in case he or she gets lost.

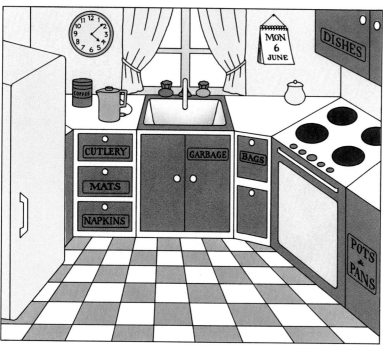

Aids to memory
Make sure that clocks and calendars can be seen easily. Make clear signs, using both words and drawings, to indicate rooms and contents of drawers, closets, and cabinets. Draw the person's attention to these memory aids as often as possible.

Communication problems

You can help the dementia sufferer communicate by ensuring that hearing aids, eyeglasses, and dentures are in place and working. Speak to the person clearly and slowly, with simple words and phrases. When talking about something in the past, make sure that the person does not confuse it with the present. Don't go along with the person's confused thinking. Correct it tactfully or change the subject. Answer repeated questions with as much consideration and patience as possible. Tell the dementia sufferer what is going on and what will be happening next, repeating information if necessary. Remind the person of the day, place, and time of year frequently. Talk about current events as a way of orienting him or her to daily life. As far as possible, allow the person to do what he or she enjoys, but make sure that dangerous situations, like crossing a busy street, are avoided.

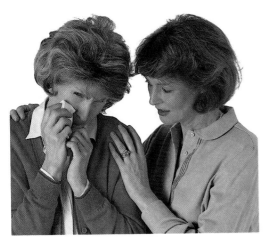

Emotional outbursts
Coping with the dementia sufferer's extreme reactions to fairly ordinary events can be difficult. Keep calm. The situation will subside more quickly than if you react strongly. Try not to take aggression or irritability personally. Remember that the person has a mental disorder. Whenever possible, avoid subjects and situations that challenge the person's memory.

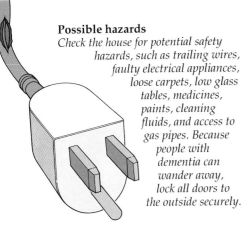

Possible hazards
Check the house for potential safety hazards, such as trailing wires, faulty electrical appliances, loose carpets, low glass tables, medicines, paints, cleaning fluids, and access to gas pipes. Because people with dementia can wander away, lock all doors to the outside securely.

CARING FOR THE CAREGIVER

If you care for someone with dementia, seek all available financial and practical help. Your local chapter of the National Alzheimer's Association will be able to provide advice. Housekeeping services, adult day-care services, home health aides, and home meal delivery may be available in your community. A variety of programs in many states give families some relief from the burden of constant care. Some programs even provide temporary boarding care.

NURSING HOME PLACEMENT

As hard as it may be, the caregiver may eventually have to acknowledge that he or she can no longer cope with or provide the necessary care for the dementia sufferer in the advanced stages of the illness. This is especially true if the caregiver is an elderly spouse or a daughter or son with a young family. The person may need constant, 24-hour care, which can be provided only in a nursing home. A social worker can help you choose a good home.

Your emotional needs

Caring for someone with dementia is physically, mentally, and emotionally draining. Do not neglect your own needs. Make sure that you take time off occasionally. Go into another room and read or just sit quietly for a while, engaged in a task that you enjoy. When possible, arrange to take a few hours off from your caregiver duties. Don't keep the situation a secret; share it with a friend. Just talking can help, and you may be surprised and gratified by the support and understanding you receive.

Find out about local groups that provide emotional support to the families of dementia patients. A support group can help you deal with negative emotions, such as anger and guilt, in an uncritical environment. Some groups organize a rotating care system to help make attendance possible. It's important to know that help is there when you need it.

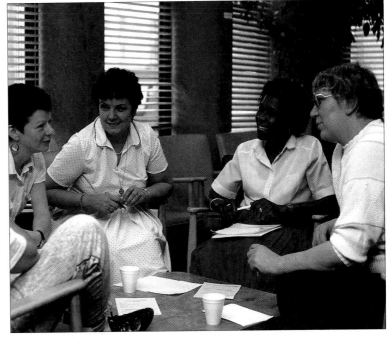

Support for the caregiver
A local support group can be vital for the caregiver's mental and emotional health. The group also serves as a source of practical advice and help.

GLOSSARY OF TERMS

Terms in *italics* in this glossary refer to other terms in the glossary.

A

Afferent
Describes a nerve that carries impulses from an organ or tissue toward the central nervous system, usually a *sensory nerve.*

Alexia
An inability to interpret the written word.

Amnesia
Loss of memory.

Amygdala
Part of the *limbic system,* which is involved with the control of behavior.

Analgesia
Loss of sensation of pain.

Anesthesia
Complete loss of sensation, also used to describe unconsciousness caused by certain drugs.

Aneurysm
Ballooning of a segment of an artery caused by an area of weakness in its wall.

Aphasia
Loss of language skills, caused by cerebral dysfunction.

Arachnoid
The middle layer of the *meninges,* the three membranes that surround and protect the brain and spinal cord.

Astrocyte
A type of *glial cell* found in the brain.

Ataxia
A disorder of muscular coordination.

Automatism
An automatic unconscious action, usually learned behavior, that is not a *reflex.*

Autonomic nervous system
The part of the nervous system responsible for many unconscious, vital functions, such as breathing and heart rate.

Axon
The extending part of a nerve cell that carries impulses away from the nerve cell body.

B

Basal ganglia
Gray matter involved with coordination of movement.

Blood-brain barrier
The cellular and biochemical barrier that prevents certain substances in the circulation from entering the brain tissues.

Brain stem
The lowest part of the brain comprised of the *midbrain,* the *pons,* and the *medulla.*

Broca's area
An area of the *cerebral cortex* that regulates speech.

C

Cerebellum
A part of the brain that controls balance and coordinated movement.

Cerebral cortex
The outer layer of *gray matter* of the *cerebrum* that controls the higher functions of the brain.

Cerebrospinal fluid
The fluid within and around the brain and spinal cord that provides support and nutrition.

Cerebrovascular accident
Stroke.

Cerebrum
The two cerebral hemispheres, each consisting of the *cerebral cortex, white matter,* and subcortical *gray matter,* that control the higher functions of the brain.

Circle of Willis
The interconnections of the major blood vessels at the base of the brain.

Coma
A state of unconsciousness in which there is little or no response to external stimulation.

Computed tomography scanning
See *CT scanning.*

Concussion
Brief loss of consciousness and function caused by head injury.

Convulsion
Seizure.

Corpus callosum
The *white matter* that connects the two cerebral hemispheres.

Cranial nerve
A nerve that arises from the brain rather than from the spinal cord.

CT (computed tomography) scanning
A diagnostic imaging technique in which X-ray beams passed through the body are detected and analyzed by a computer to produce cross-sectional images of body structures.

D

Dendrite
The short threadlike extension of a *neuron,* or nerve cell, that receives chemical signals from other *neurons.*

Dermatome
An area of skin supplied by the nerves that arise from a segment of the spinal cord.

Dura mater
The outermost layer of the three *meninges,* the protective membranes that surround the brain and spinal cord.

Dyslexia
A learning disability that affects reading and writing.

E-F

Efferent
Describes a tract or nerve that conveys impulses away from the brain or spinal cord to the muscles or glands.

Encephalitis
Inflammation of the brain, resulting from viral infection.

Frontal lobe
The part of the brain that regulates movement and elaborates thoughts.

G

Ganglion
A group of *neurons.*

Glial cell
A connective-tissue cell of the central nervous system.

Gray matter
The gray portion of the brain and spinal cord that is composed of *neuron* bodies.

Gyrus
An elevation of the surface of the brain caused by infolding of the *cerebral cortex.*

H

Hemiparesis
Partial *paralysis* that affects one side of the body.

Hemiplegia
Complete *paralysis* that affects one side of the body.

Hippocampus
Part of the *limbic system* thought to control memory.

Hydrocephalus
Excessive accumulation of *cerebrospinal fluid* inside the ventricles (cavities) of the brain.

Hypothalamus
A small structure at the base of the brain that activates, controls, and integrates the *autonomic nervous system,* the hormonal system, water intake, body temperature, sleep, food intake, and the development of the secondary sexual characteristics.

I-L

Infarct
Death of tissue due to loss of blood supply.

Limbic system
A primitive part of the brain that controls emotions and instincts and perceives odors.

M

Magnetic resonance imaging
See *MRI.*

Medulla
The lower portion of the *brain stem* that controls breathing, blood pressure, and other vital functions.

Meninges
The three membranes that surround, nourish, and protect the brain and spinal cord.

Meningitis
Inflammation of the *meninges*, usually by bacteria but sometimes by a viral infection.

Midbrain
The portion of the brain located at the top of the *brain stem* beneath the *thalamus* and surrounded by the two cerebral hemispheres.

Motor nerve
A nerve that carries impulses that cause a muscle contraction.

MRI (magnetic resonance imaging)
A diagnostic technique based on the detection of signals emitted by the nuclei of atoms inside the body when they are displaced by radio waves in a powerful magnetic field.

Myelitis
Inflammation of the spinal cord.

N

Narcolepsy
A condition characterized by sudden uncontrollable episodes of sleep, which occur at intervals.

Neocortex
The most highly evolved part of the *cerebral cortex*.

Nerve cell
See *neuron*.

Neuralgia
Pain in a nerve or the area supplied by a nerve.

Neural tube
The part of the embryo that develops into the spinal cord and brain.

Neuritis
Inflammation of a nerve.

Neuron
A nerve cell, composed of a cell body, branching projections called *dendrites*, and an extended fiber (*axon*) that conducts impulses.

Neurotransmitter
A chemical released by a nerve ending at a *synapse*, which binds with a *receptor* on the target tissue to produce a response.

Nystagmus
A rhythmic jerking movement of the eyes that occurs in certain neurological disorders or that sometimes occurs in healthy people.

O-P

Ophthalmoplegia
Paralysis of the eye muscles.

Palsy
Paralysis.

Paralysis
The loss of nerve impulses to a muscle, resulting in an inability to use that muscle.

Paraplegia
Total *paralysis* of the lower extremities.

Parasympathetic nervous system
The part of the *autonomic nervous system* that predominates during times of relaxation. It conserves and restores energy.

Paresis
Incomplete *paralysis*.

Paresthesia
A sensory disturbance that produces a prickly feeling of "pins and needles."

PET (positron emission tomography) scanning
An imaging technique based on the detection of particles emitted when radioactive substances are introduced into the body.

Photophobia
Abnormal intolerance to light.

Pia mater
The inner layer of the *meninges*.

Pineal gland
A tiny part of the brain thought to be involved in the control of daily biological cycles.

Pituitary gland
The gland attached to the *hypothalamus* that produces many hormones to control the endocrine system and other functions.

Plexus
A network of interwoven nerves.

Pons
The middle portion of the *brain stem*.

Positron emission tomography
See *PET scanning*.

Proprioception
The sense (awareness) of position and movement.

Q-R

Quadriplegia
Complete *paralysis* of the trunk and all four limbs

Receptor
A specific molecule on the surface of or within a cell to which a *neurotransmitter*, hormone, or other chemical binds to produce a physiological effect. In the case of nerve cells, the effect is the creation and transmission of an impulse along the nerve, or the stimulation of a target tissue.

Reflex
An unlearned involuntary response to a stimulus.

S

Seizure
A sudden episode of abnormal brain activity resulting in loss of consciousness or involuntary movements or behaviors.

Sensory nerve
A nerve that carries information regarding the senses.

Spasm
A sudden, involuntary, painful muscle contraction that interferes with normal function.

Spasticity
Increased rigidity in a group of muscles that causes stiffness and restriction of movement.

Status epilepticus
A series of rapidly repeating *seizures* with no intervals of consciousness.

Stroke
Localized damage to the brain caused by a burst or blocked blood vessel, often resulting in physical disability and/or mental impairment.

Sulcus
An infolding or creased area of the *cerebral cortex*.

Sympathetic nervous system
The part of the *autonomic nervous system* that predominates at times of stress. Its actions tend to cause energy expenditure.

Synapse
The junction between one *neuron* and another into which *neurotransmitters* are released.

T

Temporal lobe
The lower side lobe of the cerebral hemisphere that perceives sounds and odors and controls some language functions and some functions of the *limbic system*.

Tetany
Sudden *spasm* of muscles caused by abnormal neuromuscular response to bacterial toxins, low blood levels of calcium or magnesium, and other factors.

Thalamus
A gray structure deep within the brain that relays sensory signals from lower brain structures to the *cerebral cortex* and performs other functions.

Tic
An involuntary repetitive movement usually involving the muscles of the face and shoulder.

Tinnitus
A ringing sound in the ears.

Tract
A collection or bundle of nerve fibers, usually quite long, that have the same origin, destination, and function.

Tremor
Involuntary trembling.

V-W

Ventricle
A natural cavity inside the brain filled with *cerebrospinal fluid*.

Vertigo
A spinning sensation.

Wernicke's area
An area of the *cerebral cortex* that interprets sensory information and language functions.

White matter
The white portion of the brain and spinal cord, composed of nerve fibers and connective tissue but no cell bodies.

Photograph sources:
Art Directors Photo Library **77**; **83**
St. Bartholomews Hospital **93**; **124** (top left)
Biophoto Associates **45**
Blackwells Scientific publishing **111**; **131**
(bottom left)
Collections **41** (top right)
Dr Daniels, The Brain Bank **116**
Bruce Coleman Ltd **75** (top left)
Mary Evans Picture Library **25** (top left); **79**
Sally and Richard Greenhill **139**
The Image Bank **7**; **39**; **63**; **67**
Magnum **128** (top left)
St. Mary's Hospital **124** (bottom right)
National Medical Slide Bank, UK **131** (top
left)
Ann and Bury Peerless **41** (top left)
Pictor International **51**; **102**; **122** (bottom
right)

Rex Features **65**
Science Photo Library **2** (bottom right) **9**; **19**;
21; **25** (center); **27**; **37**; **44**; **52**; **90**; **98**; **99**; **107**;
114 (bottom right); **128** (top right, bot-
tom); **129** (top left); **134**; **135**
Dr J.B.P. Stephenson **95**
Tony Stone Worldwide **97**; **114** (top center)
Transport and Road Research Laboratory
122 (bottom left)
Dr I. Williams **129** (bottom right)
Zefa **2** (top left); **41** (bottom right)
Front cover photograph: Luis Castaneda/
The Image Bank

**'Medic Alert' is a registered trademark of
the Medic Alert Foundation**

Index:
Sue Bosanko

Illustrators:
Karen Cochrane
David Fathers
Tony Graham
Andrew Green
Coral Mula
Gilly Newman
Philip Wilson
John Woodcock

Airbrushing:
Paul Desmond
Roy Flooks
Janos Marffy

**Commissioned
photography:**
Susannah Price
Steve Bartholomew